5 Ingredients or less Keto Diet Air Fryer Cookbook

Top 99 Quick, Easy and Delicious Low Carb Ketogenic Diet Air Fryer Recipes to Save Time and Money, Lose Weight Fast and Upgrade Your Lifestyle

By Jalan Rashid

© **Copyright 2018 -Jalan Rashid-All rights reserved.**

In no way is it legal to reproduce, duplicate, or transmit any part of this document by either electronic means or in printed format. Recording of this publication is strictly prohibited, and any storage of this material is not allowed unless with written permission from the publisher. All rights reserved.

The information provided herein is stated to be truthful and consistent, in that any liability, regarding inattention or otherwise, by any usage or abuse of any policies, processes, or directions contained within is the solitary and complete responsibility of the recipient reader. Under no circumstances will any legal liability or blame be held against the publisher for any reparation, damages, or monetary loss due to the information herein, either directly or indirectly.

Respective authors own all copyrights not held by the publisher.

Legal Notice:
This book is copyright protected. This is only for personal use. You cannot amend, distribute, sell, use, quote or paraphrase any part or the content within this book without the consent of the author or copyright owner. Legal action will be pursued if this is breached.

Table of Contents

Introduction 7
Chapter 1: Ketogenic Diet Basics 8

    What is Ketogenic Diet? 8
    How the Keto Diet Works 8
    What is Exactly Ketosis? 8
    Optimal conditions for Keeping Ketosis 9
    Some Unwanted Symptoms to recognize during Ketosis 10
    The Difference Between Ketogenic Diet and Low Carb Diet 10
    Amazing Keto Food List 11
    Easy-To-Get Keto Advantages You Must Know 13
    Is Keto Really Suitable For Someone With Diabetes? 14
    Can Keto Help Lose Weight Faster? 14
    Most Useful Tips and Tricks For A Keto Journey 14

Chapter 2: Air Fryer 101 16

    What is an Air Fryer? 16
    Looking at the individual components of Air Fryer 17
    Common Features of Air Fryer 19
    Benefits of Air Fryer Cooking 19
    Keeping your device clean 20
    Easy and Simple steps for using an Air Fryer 20
    Cooking Time of Various Foods 21
    Choosing Your Right Fryer 24
    Pros and Cons of the Air Fryer 26
    Top 3 Air Fryers As Your Choice 26

Chapter 3: Chicken And Poultry 29

    Cheesy Drumsticks 29
    Crunchy Chicken Skin 30
    Chicken Scallops 31
    Chicken Skewers 32
    Country Chicken 33
    Ginger Chicken Thighs 34
    Lime Chicken 35
    Schnitzel Parmigiana 36
    Cheesy Chicken Bites 37

Jerk Chicken Wings 38

Chapter 4: Pork, Beef, Lamb **39**

Beef Tongue 39
Pork Rinds 40
Ribeye Steak 41
Pork Chops 42
Parmesan Beef 43
Roast Beef 44
Fried Lamb Chops 44
Pork Roast 45
T-Bone 46
Bacon wrapped Asparagus Spears 47
Fried Italian Meatballs 48
Cheese And Ham Pinwheels 49
Bacon Cabbage 50
Bacon Brussel Sprouts 51

Chapter 5: Fish And Seafood **52**

Spicy Garlic Shrimp...52
Butter And Garlic Salmon 53
Bacon Wrapped Shrimp 54
Cajun Shrimp 55
Smoked Trout Frittata 56
Pineapple Ham Steak 57
Fried Cod 58
Crab Sticks 58
Fish Nuggets 59
Squid Rings 60
Almond Crusted Halibut 61
Catfish 62

Chapter 6: Vegan And Vegetarian **63**

Buffalo Cauliflower 63
Apple Chips 64
Fried Dill Pickles 65
Avocado Fries 66
Fried Brussel Sprouts 67

Winter Veggies 68
Roasted Carrots 69
Banana Chips 69
Garlic Green Peppers 70
Curried Cauliflower 70
Stuffed Peppers 71
Fried Pumpkin Seeds 72
Fried Parsnips 73
Kale Chips 74
Spicy Asparagus 75
Zucchini Gratin 76
Spaghetti Squash 77
Cabbage Steaks 78
Eggplant Parmesan 79
Green and Yellow Beans 80
Tofu 81
Zucchini Zoodles 82
Onion Rings 83
Turnips 84
Radish Chips 85

Chapter 7: Appetizers 86

Bread 86
Scrambled Eggs 87
Egg Soufflé 87
Cheesy Sweet Potatoes 88
Vegetable Parmesan Bites 89
Carrot Fries 90
Cheesy Broccoli 91
Portobello Pizza 92
Cheddar Bacon Croquettes 93
Crispy Shirataki Noodles 94
Spinach Chips 95
Siracha Shrimp 96
Daikon Fries 97
Egg Clouds 98
Egg Soufflé 99
Spam Fries 99
Buffalo Wings 100

Stuffed Mushrooms 101
Keto-Friendly Bacon 102
Cheese bites 103
Chicken Livers 104
Fried Eggs 105
Grilled Cheese 105
Chicken Strips 106
Brisket Bites 107
Zucchini Fries 108
Fried Okra 109
Bacon Wrapped Jalapenos 110
Onion And Sage Stuffed Balls 111
Warm Broccoli Salad 112
Egg Tarts 113
Parmesan Sticks 114

Chapter 8: Desserts 115

Apricot And Blackberry Crumble 115
Fried Pineapple 116
Toasted Marshmallows 116
Banana Fritters 117
Vanilla Custard 118
Mini chocolate cake 119

Conclusion 120

Introduction

Let me start by thanking you for taking the time to purchase this book.

While writing this book, my core aim was to ensure that readers were able to easily grasp the concept of Ketogenic Diet and the Air Fryer. I tried my very best to keep this book as easy to understand as possible.

The book has been divided into chapters; which are then divided into bite-sized sections focusing on a single topic.

The first chapter explains the ins and outs of Ketogenic Diet, while the second chapter provides the basics to properly use your Air Fryer.

Once you are done exploring the early chapters of the book, you will be able to enjoy 100 Ketogenic Air Fryer recipes.

I hope you enjoy the book and Ketogenic Diet while using your Air Fryer to the fullest extent.

Happy Cooking!

Chapter 1: Ketogenic Diet Basics

What is Ketogenic Diet?

When considering Ketogenic Diet, typically the first thing that comes to mind is, "What does Keto mean?"

Well, the word Keto is derived from a natural, human metabolic process known as Ketosis; allowing your body to generate a chemical substance known as Ketones.

The core objective of Ketogenic Diet is to lower your carb intake to allow your body to increase the production of Ketones, and maintain a state of Ketosis.

How the Keto Diet Works

That being said, to fully understand and appreciate the working process of Ketogenic Diet, you must first learn that when your body is exposed to a high amount of carbohydrates, it tends to increase the production of glucose and insulin.

Glucose; being the converting molecule in our body, it is the body's first choice when considering a chemical to break down and produce energy for the body.

Here's the thing. When glucose is abundantly present in our body, it significantly decreases the amount of fat burned through working out or dieting, since the body tends to burn reserved glucose instead of fat.

This is a very important point and also one of the main reasons why some people tend to work really hard and get no result in the long run.

And this is exactly where the Ketogenic Diet saves the day.

When you cut off the carbohydrate intake to your body, it slowly starts to enter a state known as Ketosis; which is basically the body's natural response kicking in when it senses low carb intake.

What is Exactly Ketosis?

As already mentioned, the core objective of the Ketogenic Diet is to allow an individual to enter into a state of Ketosis.

Simply put, when you are cutting down the intake of carbohydrates from your daily routine, your body starts to burn fat instead of carbohydrates.

This fat burning process is further accelerated due to the release of chemicals known as Ketones, as they further force the body to break down fat instead of glucose.
This whole process is known as Ketosis.

Optimal conditions for Keeping Ketosis

While the exact conditions for an individual to maintain Ketosis will vary, the following rule of thumb will help you accelerate the process of achieving and maintaining a Keto state.

Reducing carb intake will have the highest impact, there are a few more steps to follow to improve the process:

- Keep daily carbohydrate intake below 20g carbs.
- Keep protein levels at around 70g per day.
- Don't starve. Consume adequate amount of fat. Remember the body needs fat to burn fat.
- Avoid snacking; stick to breakfast, lunch, and dinner meals with nothing in between.

Some tips you should be aware of:

- **Frequent desire to urinate:** Ketosis will cause your body to burn up more fat; glycogen is stored. Kidneys start to process more water, increasing your urge to urinate.
- **Hypoglycemia:** Sugar level reduced.
- **Constipation:** Possible side effect due to dehydration and reduced salt in the body. Easily rectified by drinking more water.
- **Increased Sugar Craving:** May experience craving for sugar. To tackle this, you can supplement your diet with extra protein and vitamin B complex. A good, brisk walk works as well.
- **Diarrhea:** Common issue faced by some people during the first few days, but it resolves itself after a few days. It's like flushing out all the toxins.
- **Sleep problem:** This can be a result of reduced levels of serotonin or insulin. Should settle down.

Most of these issues can be rectified by increased water consumption.

Some Unwanted Symptoms to recognize during Ketosis

Now that you have a good idea of Ketosis, these are symptoms you should keep an eye out for in the early days of your journey.

While there are various advanced techniques, such as using a urine strip to check your Ketone level, you can assess it by observing the following indicators:

- Dry mouth, and increased thirst.
- Frequent washroom visits; urge to urinate more often.
- Breath will have a slight fruity smell; resembling that of nail polish.
- Experience low hunger level; increased energy.

The Difference Between Ketogenic Diet and Low Carb Diet

There are some people out there who often mistake certain aspects of a low-carb diet as Ketogenic and ultimately follow a low-carb diet while claiming they are following a Keto diet.

This is pretty normal as there are subtle, yet crucial differences between the two; everyone is not aware of these.

I will try to clarify the differences between the two.

These low carb diets often allow for 50-150 grams of carbs per day, however, there are some athletes who prefer to consume a HIGH low-carb diet that allows for 200g per day due to greater caloric requirement.

Ketogenic on the other hand is much more formulated, and well-designed compared to low-carb diet that follows a very precise dietary regime calling for high-fat, moderate protein, and low-carb approach.

A typical Ketogenic diet will allow you to consume 20-50 grams of carbs per day and the macronutrient profile will call for a daily meal plan that is made up of 20% protein, 5% carbs and 75% fat.

This different macronutrient profile is designed in such a way that allows your body to start using ketones as an alternate fuel source for energy that exponentially increases fat burning process in the body.

Amazing Keto Food List

Fat:

Recommend

- Saturated Fat; coconut oil ghee
- Monosaturated Fat; olive, macadamia, almond oil
- Polyunsaturated Omega 3; sardines
- Medium Chain Triglycerides; fatty acid
- Lard
- Chicken Fat
- Duck Fat
- Goose Fat

Avoid

- Refined Fats and Oils; sunflower, soybean, corn oil
- Trans Fat; margarine

Protein:

Recommend

- Grass fed meat
- Harvested seafood and wild caught meat
- Free-range organic eggs
- Beef
- Lamb
- Goat
- Venison
- Pastured Pork
- Poultry

Avoid

- Factory packed animal foods and produce

Vegetables:

Recommend

- Leafy green vegetables
- Low carb vegetables

- Swiss chard
- Bok Choy
- Lettuce
- Chard
- Chives
- Endives
- Radicchio

Avoid

- High starch = high carb vegetables; peas, potatoes, yucca, beans, legumes

Dairy Products:
Recommend

- Dairy products; yogurt, sour cream, cottage cheese, goat cheese, whole milk

Avoid

- Low fat/ Skim Milk

Fruits:
Recommend

- In general, choose fruits that are low carb and have more fat; berries, avocados

Avoid

- Try to avoid dried fruits; they high in sugar content

Drinks
Recommend

- Water
- Black Coffee
- Unsweetened and Herbal Teas
- Nut Milks
- Light Beets
- Wine

Avoid

- Soft Drinks; Pepsi or Coke

- High Fructose Syrup
- Nectar
- Honey

Sweeteners

Recommend

- Stevia
- Xylitol
- Erythritol
- Inulin
- Monk Fruit Powder
- Dark Chocolate Cocoa

Easy-To-Get Keto Advantages You Must Know

Looking at the avoid food list might discourage you but the advantages far outweigh the demerits of the diet.

- ✓ The diet will help reduce bad cholesterol levels and prevent arterial blockings.
- ✓ Energy from burning fat will keep your body energized due to the presence of good fat in your body.
- ✓ The LDL levels will decrease, in turn reducing your chance of suffering from Type-2 Diabetes.
- ✓ Control your hunger and appetite.
- ✓ Skin appearance will improve and help prevent skin inflammation and acne.

But what about other benefits of Ketogenic Diet?

- Keto will also directly help increase the amount of fat burnt through daily activities.
- Consume a significant amount of protein that will contribute to weight loss.
- Once you have reduced bad carbohydrates, calorie intake will diminish and contribute to increased weight loss.
- Gluconeogenesis will start to cause your body to burn more fat.

Is Keto Really Suitable For Someone With Diabetes?

It has been observed that people who are obese can dramatically reduce their chances of developing diabetes by eating a balanced and nutritious diet.

Following a diet full of vitamins and minerals and low in added sugar and unhealthy fat helps individuals to lose extra fat.

That being said, it has also been seen that people who lose 5-10% of their body weight can reduce their risk of diabetes by about 58%.

That is huge if you think about it.

For people who are already suffering from diabetes, losing the same amount of weight will help to bring the blood sugar under control as well.

Since a core aspect of the Ketogenic diet is to help you to lose weight through Ketosis, Ketogenic diet also indirectly helps to control diabetes while helping lower blood glucose levels.

Can Keto Help Lose Weight Faster?

One of the main reasons you are reading this book is for assistance losing weight. Well, the good news is that Keto diet will help you burn fat quickly!

When you start to eat more carbs, your body burns carbs instead of fat in order to produce energy for the body.

However, when you remove carbohydrates from the equation, the stored glycogen will eventually burn out and the body will start to burn fat in order to get energy.

This does not only help you to burn fat, but it also helps you to burn triglycerides that are stored in your body as fatty cells.

All of these effects together, result in your body shrinking fat cells, eventually making you leaner and less obese.

Most Useful Tips and Tricks For A Keto Journey

Some good pointers for a Keto-friendly journey include:

- Get yourself a carb counter to keep your daily carb intake in check.
- Make sure to get rid of all of the high-carb products from your kitchen.
- Slowly try to alter your daily habits and accept new ones in order to make sure they complement your new life style.
- Stay as hydrated as you can by drinking water.

- Keep sodium intake in check; will make your Keto journey more pleasant. You can do this by:
    - ✓ Drinking organic broth, if possible.
    - ✓ Including a pinch of pink salt with your meals.
    - ✓ Adding vegetables; kelp, cucumber, celery for a more natural approach to sodium replenishment.
- Include a basic amount of physical exercise in your diet regime. It would not only make you healthy, but accelerate the effectiveness of your Keto diet.
    - ✓ A general exercise routine may include:
        - ❖ Monday: Resistance training for upper body; 20 minutes.
        - ❖ Tuesday: Resistance training for Lower Body; 20 minutes.
        - ❖ Wednesday: Long walk; 30 minutes.
        - ❖ Thursday: Resistance training for upper body; 20 minutes.
        - ❖ Friday: Resistance training for Lower Body; 20 minutes.
        - ❖ Sat/Sun: Recreational time.

Chapter 2: Air Fryer 101

Generally speaking, the technology used in the Air Fryer is still relatively new when compared with other more well-known kitchen appliances. While the device has already penetrated into the kitchens of thousands around the world, there is still a large chunk of people who are unaware of this technological marvel.

If you are one of them, this is the time for you to get to know the true potential of the Air Fryer and learn how to appreciate this amazing device.

What is an Air Fryer?

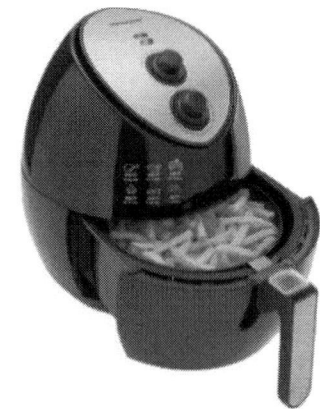

You may have seen different advertisements trying to explain how Air Fryer is a wonderful device that seamlessly utilizes hot air to cook food.

The advertisers are right; there is little more to an Air Fryer than simply that.

A fantastic, modern piece of kitchen equipment that not only helps to make one's life easier, but also elevate his lifestyle by providing a healthier food palate that minimizes the use of oil.

In fact, the popularity of oil-free cooking and the air fryer device itself has reached such high levels that Gordon Ramsey claimed, 'Air is the new oil.'

The mechanism

But how does the Air Fryer actually work you might wonder?

Well. The answer actually lies in the way the Air Fryer prepares the meals.

While most cooking appliances tend to rely on traditional cooking methods, such as conduction heating, the Air Fryer does a phenomenal job of going against the regular trend and utilizing the technique of convection heating.

The "Air" is responsible for the magic here! Back when this technology was introduced to the market, it was met with massive critical reception that to this day, does not fail to impress budding chefs around the world.

Rapid Air Technology; delicately designed process which the Air Fryer uses to cook its food.

Upon sucking up the air into its intake chamber, the appliance immediately cranks up the heat and raises the temperature of the air inside. The air is then passed through a specialized cooking cell, where the meal is prepared and cooked. This whole process is the mechanism behind the term rapid air technology.

Perhaps the biggest benefit of this is thanks to the use of "Air." The appliance is able to cook meals without using oil, or greatly minimizing the amount of oil used.

This not only helps to boast a healthier lifestyle, but complements the Ketogenic diet.

Looking at the individual components of Air Fryer

If you are a completely new user of the Air Fryer, the various parts of the fryer might confuse you at first. However, this section will help you to clear up any confusion you may have by giving you a brief overview of the individual components.

In general, an Air Fryer consists of:

- **Cook Chamber:** Chamber of the fryer where the actual cooking takes place. It should be noted that the cook chamber may vary from one brand to the next. Some Fryers might have walled cook baskets, while others have normal cook baskets.

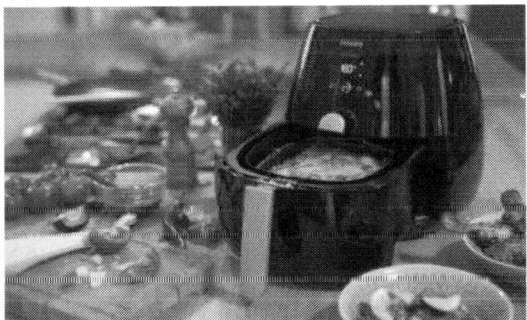

- **Heating Element:** The coil inside the fryer that produces the heat once electricity passes through it. Once the heating element reaches the desired temperature, air is passed through this coil, where it heats up and passes through the fan and grill.

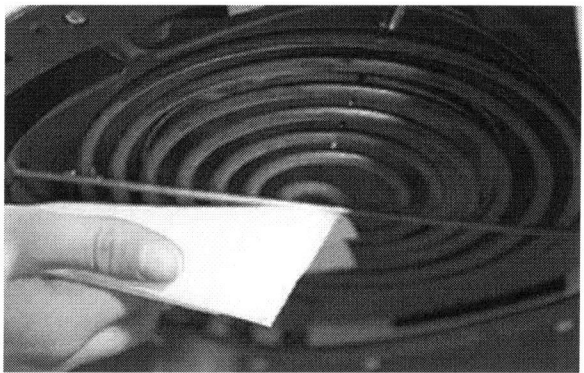

- **Fan and Grill:** The fan and grill work together to ensure everything is cooked well. These two are responsible for proper circulation of the superheated air.

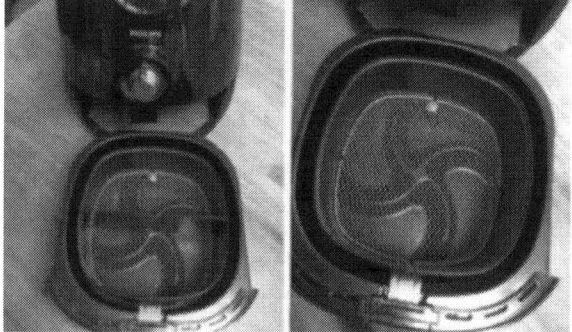

- **Exhaust System:** The exhaust system helps to release excess pressure and prevent harmful build up. Modern Air Fryers also include filters that help to get rid of dirt, and help to prevent unpleasant odors from the appliance.
- **Transferable Food Tray:** There are some brands which include several boundary walls built within the tray; allowing to cook multiple dishes. Some brands also have a universal handle; allowing to remove tray from heating chamber with ease.

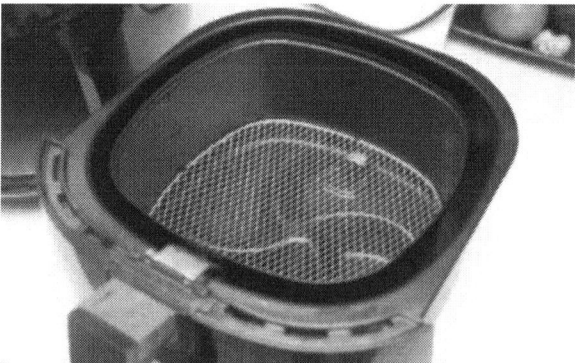

Common Features of Air Fryer

You should know that different Air Fryer companies will try to include something to make their device unique. However, the following are pretty much staple to all Air Fryers out there:

- **Automated Temperature Control System:** Optimal temperature levels throughout cook session to ensure even cooking.
- **Digital Screen and Touch Panel:** Easily control device and seamlessly alter settings without hassle.
- **Convenient Buzzer:** Won't have to stand in front of the device to make sure your meals are not burnt.
- **Assorted Selection of Cook Presets:** Multiple pre-set cook settings. You won't have to worry about setting the time or temperature, as optimal parameters already set for you.

PRESET BUTTON COOKING CHART		
PRESET BUTTON	TEMPERATURE	TIME
French Fries	400°F	20 min
Roasts	370°F	15 min
Shrimp	330°F	15 min
Baked Goods	350°F	25 min
Chicken	380°F	25 min
Steak	380°F	25 min
Fish	390°F	25 min

Benefits of Air Fryer Cooking

Along with reducing about 80% of oil intake from your life, other advantages include:

- Air Fryer is convenient and easy to use.
- Cleaning Air Fryer is extremely easy and does not make a mess.
- Oil free meals will contribute to weight loss and improve your health.
- Air Fryer allows to cook meals rapidly.

Keeping your device clean

As human beings, we are prone to making mistakes. But knowing about the common mistakes beforehand might just save us from going through the hassle of facing such difficulties.

Some of the common mistakes newcomers tend to make while cooking with an Air Fryer:

- Make sure to give your Air Fryer sufficient room to breathe; essentially keep your Air Fryer free from cramped spaces or corners.
- Keep your Air Fryer disconnected when not in use. The Air Fryer takes minimal amount of time to heat up, so you won't have to keep it connected for a lengthy period to heat up.
- Use light baking trays or dishes; dark material can absorb more heat. This may result in uneven cooking.

Some additional tips when cleaning:

- ✓ Soak in warm water and mild dish detergent before cleaning to increase optimal cleaning.
- ✓ When cleaning your Air Fryer, use simple cloths or sponges as metal parts of the appliance can scratch easily.

Easy and Simple steps for using an Air Fryer

Using an Air Fryer is pretty simple.

- If using oil, lightly spray the cook basket or the food; will avoid food sticking.
- Even if spraying with oil, pat dry any excess liquid so fryer doesn't smoke while cooking.
- Shake the food gently after 5 minutes of cooking for even cooking
- Prepare ingredients of the meal according to directions.
- Transfer prepared tray to cook basket, and follow instructions.
- If baking a cake, pour batter in separate dish and place on cook tray.
- Set temperature to specified temperature and set timer.
- Cook times are a guide. It is recommended to test what works best for your recipes.

- Most recipes will require little to no oil; overall oil intake will be reduced by almost 80%.
- Clean oil catch of fryer frequently; for optimal cooking results.

Cooking Time of Various Foods

The following is a list of preparation and cook times for common items.

- ✓ **Thick Frozen Fries**
  Minimum Amount: 2 cups
  Maximum Amount: 4 cups
  Cook time: 12 – 22 minutes
  Temperature: 360°F
  Halfway Point Shake: Yes
  Extra Remarks: Spray lightly with non-stick Keto cooking spray. Season with preferred spices at halfway point.

- ✓ **Thin Frozen Fries**
  Minimum Amount: 2 cups
  Maximum Amount: 4 cups
  Cook time: 9 – 19 minutes
  Temperature: 360°F
  Halfway Point Shake: Yes
  Extra Remarks: Spray lightly with non-stick Keto cooking spray. Season with preferred spices at halfway point.

- ✓ **Fresh Homemade Fries**
  Minimum Amount: 2 cups
  Maximum Amount: 4 cups
  Cook time: 15 – 22 minutes
  Temperature: 360°F
  Halfway Point Shake: Yes
  Extra Remarks: For crispy consistency: Soak fries in cold water 30 minutes (change water twice). Pat dry well. Spray lightly with non-stick Keto cooking spray. Season with preferred spices.

- ✓ **Fresh Potato Wedges**
  Minimum Amount: 2 cups
  Maximum Amount: 4 cups
  Cook time: 18 – 21 minutes
  Temperature: 360°F
  Halfway Point Shake: Yes
  Extra Remarks: For crispy consistency: Soak wedges in cold water 30 minutes (change water twice). Pat dry well. Spray lightly with non-stick Keto cooking spray. Season with preferred spices.

- ✓ **Fresh Potato Cubes**
  Minimum Amount: 2 cups
  Maximum Amount: 4 cups
  Cook time: 18 – 21 minutes
  Temperature: 360°F
  Halfway Point Shake: Yes
  Extra Remarks: For crispy consistency: Soak cubes in cold water 30 minutes (change water twice). Pat dry well. Spray lightly with non-stick Keto cooking spray. Season with preferred spices.

- ✓ **Fresh Cheese Sticks**
  Minimum Amount: 6 pieces
  Maximum Amount: 12 pieces
  Cook time: 8 – 10 minutes
  Temperature: 360°F
  Halfway Point Shake: Yes
  Extra Remarks: Spray lightly with non-stick Keto cooking spray.

- ✓ **Frozen Cheese Sticks**
  Minimum Amount: 6 pieces
  Maximum Amount: 12 pieces
  Cook time: 9 – 19 minutes
  Temperature: 360°F
  Halfway Point Shake: Yes
  Extra Remarks: Spray lightly with non-stick Keto cooking spray.

- ✓ **Frozen Chicken Nuggets**
  Minimum Amount: 6 pieces
  Maximum Amount: 12 pieces
  Cook time: 6 – 10 minutes
  Temperature: 390°F
  Halfway Point Shake: Yes
  Extra Remarks: Spray lightly with non-stick Keto cooking spray.

- ✓ **Frozen Fish Sticks**
  Minimum Amount: 6 pieces
  Maximum Amount: 12 pieces
  Cook time: 8 – 10 minutes
  Temperature: 390°F
  Halfway Point Shake: Yes
  Extra Remarks: Spray lightly with non-stick Keto cooking spray.

- ✓ **Steak**
  Minimum Amount: 4 ounce piece
  Maximum Amount: 8 ounce piece
  Cook time: Depending on desired doneness. Cook according to your preference.
  4 ounce piece – cook 4 minutes at 360°F, followed by 4 minutes at 150°F.
  8 ounce piece – cook 6 minutes at 360°F, followed by 6 minutes at 150°F.
  Temperature: Start: 360°F, Finish: 150°F
  Halfway Point Shake: No
  Extra Remarks: Spray lightly with non-stick Keto cooking spray. Season with preferred spices.

- ✓ **Hamburger patties**
  Minimum Amount: 2 medium patties (increase cooking time with thickness)
  Maximum Amount: 4 medium patties (increase cooking time with thickness)
  Cook time: 6 – 7 minutes
  Temperature: 360°F
  Halfway Point Shake: No
  Extra Remarks: Spray lightly with non-stick Keto cooking spray. Season with preferred spices.

- ✓ **Fresh Chicken Wings**
  Minimum Amount: 6 pieces
  Maximum Amount: 12 pieces
  Cook time: 18 – 22 minutes
  Temperature: 360°F
  Halfway Point Shake: No
  Extra Remarks: Spray lightly with non-stick Keto cooking spray. Season with preferred spices.

- ✓ **Fresh Chicken Breast**
  Minimum Amount: 4 ounce piece
  Maximum Amount: 8 ounce piece
  Cook time: 4 ounce piece – cook 4 minutes at 290°F, followed by 4 minutes at 360°F.
  8 ounce piece – cook 6 minutes at 290°F, followed by 6 minutes at 360°F.
  Temperature: Start: 290°F, Finish: 360°F
  Halfway point Shake: No
  Extra Remarks: Spray lightly with non-stick Keto cooking spray. Season with preferred spices.

- ✓ **Cake**
  Minimum Amount: 2 cups
  Maximum Amount: 4 cups
  Cook time: 18 – 30 minutes
  Temperature: 320°F
  Halfway Point Shake: No
  Extra Remarks: None

Choosing Your Right Fryer

Buying an Air Fryer might seem a little confusing at first.
I have designed this brief section, hoping it would help to select the best Air Fryer to suit your needs and give you the best bang for your buck.
Certain parameters to keep in mind when buying your Air Fryer:

- Capacity

- Accessibility
- Accessories
- Price
- Pros and Cons of the device

The ultimate decision will come down to your requirements and budget.

Capacity

You will have the choice of small or large; depending on the size of your family.
To give you an idea,

- Philips Air Fryer; capacity between 1.8 pounds to 2.6 pounds
- Tefal Actifry; capacity 2.2 pounds
- Lidore Air Fryer; 22 pound capacity
- Avalon Bay Air Fryer; capacity 3.2 pounds

Accessibility

Air Fryers generally have three different modes of operation:

- Analog button
- Digital interface with interactive touch screen
- Pre-set options

Devices with analog buttons don't have that many extra features, but get the job done just fine.

Modern Air Fryers on the other hand, such as Philips, tend to come with digital touch pad control that offers a wide range of programmable settings allowing you to modify the cooking parameters depending on your recipe.

You will also be able to use pre-set options that makes the process of cooking much easier; parameters already installed and ready to use with the touch of your finger.

Accessories

Certain options will help expand your cooking options and make your appliance even more versatile.

Accessories that you should be looking for include:

- Double Layer Rack
- Grill Pan
- Skewers
- Cake Pan

- Rotisserie Fork
- Fry Cage
- Steak Cage

It is rare you get all the accessories in a single package, therefore, it is wise to do your research and check whether the model you want comes with the accessories you need. Certain models, such as a Gourmia GTA1500 comes with 4 accessories, while the Philips Air Fryer doesn't come with a variety of accessories. Accessories can be bought separately.

When it comes to buying accessories though, brand doesn't really mean that much. Pick ones that fit easily in the Air Fryer you are using and you will be good to go.

Price

When buying your Air Fryer, it could be economical to browse the web and compare prices before choosing the model that is best for you.

Pros and Cons of the Air Fryer

Pros

- Minimal or no oil used while cooking
- Accessible and easy to use
- Cook at faster rate
- Convenient to use
- Easy to clean
- Multiple cooking modes

Cons

- Made for general use; larger meals generally require to be cooked in batches
- Device is rather bulky, needs space

Top 3 Air Fryers As Your Choice

Tefal Actifry Express XL

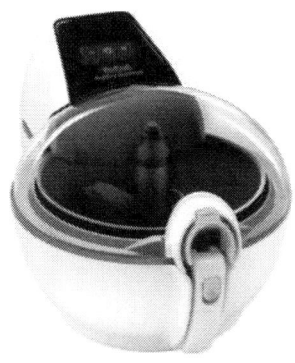

The Tefal Actifry Express XL is best for feeding a large family; able to cook about 4 pounds of food per batch. With user-friendly and easy-to-use controls, this device makes Air Fryer a breeze.
Price: 305$

Vonshef 2.2L

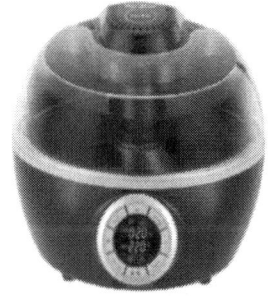

This device falls towards the bargain spectrum while not sacrificing any of the modern features. Comes with a sleek design and digital display that makes it look futuristic and accessible. Batches of 1½ pounds of food can be cooked at any given time.
Price: 77$

NuWave Brio Digital

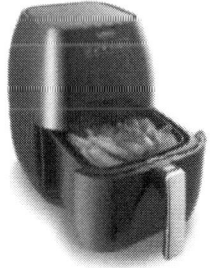

This device has made quite a name for itself in the US market. The Air Flow Technology implemented in this device is really top notch; allows food to be cooked evenly. Also, comes with a large, approximately 6 pound capacity basket; can feed a moderately big family.

Price: 172$

You are now ready to delve into the recipes.

Note 1: Most cook times are a guide; please test the recipes for optimal cook time for the amount of food and fryer you have chosen. Always make sure the food is cooked thoroughly before consuming; use a food thermometer.

Note 2: When cooking in batches, it is recommended to heat your oven to 300°F to keep cooked food warm as you fry rest of ingredients.

Note 3: Sometimes the recipe will recommend placing ingredients in freezer, it is to settle the coating.

Chapter 3: Chicken And Poultry

Cheesy Drumsticks

(Prep time: 18 minutes\ Cook time: 15 minutes\ 2 servings)

Ingredients

- 1 pound small to medium bone in chicken drumsticks (boneless, reduce cooking time)
- 2 Tbsp almond flour
- 1 cup mixed finely grated cheeses; parmesan, cheddar
- 1 tsp dried rosemary
- 1 tsp dried oregano
- ½ tsp chili flakes (optional)
- ½ tsp salt, pepper
- Garnish: chopped green onion

Directions

1. Rinse the drumsticks. Pat dry.
2. In a medium bowl, combine the flour, mixed cheeses, herbs, chili flakes, salt, pepper.
3. Dip drumsticks in mixture, turn until evenly coated. Place in freezer 5 minutes.
4. Spray chicken or fryer lightly with non-stick Keto cooking spray. Pre-heat fryer to 370°F.
5. Transfer drumsticks to fryer. Cook 15 minutes; shake at halfway point, cook thoroughly.
6. Transfer to serving plate. Garnish with chopped green onion.

Nutrition Values (Per Serving)

- Calories: 226
- Fat: 10g
- Carbohydrates: 1g
- Protein: 16g

Crunchy Chicken Skin

(Prep time: 10 minutes\ Cook time: 6 minutes\ 2 servings)

Ingredients

- 1 pound chicken skin
- 1 tsp dried dill
- ½ tsp chili flakes
- 1 tsp butter
- ½ tsp salt, pepper

Directions

1. Rinse the chicken skin. Pat dry.
2. Melt the butter. Allow to cool slightly.
3. Roughly chop chicken skin. Dip in melted butter.
4. Combine the dill, chili flakes, salt, pepper in a baggie.
5. Add the skin to baggie, shake until evenly coated.
6. Pre-heat the fryer to 360°F. Lightly spray cook basket with non-stick Keto cooking spray.
7. Transfer chicken skin to fryer. Cook 3 minutes, shake briskly. Cook 3 more minutes; until crispy.
8. Transfer to paper towel, lightly pat dry. Allow to cool 5 minutes before eating.

Nutrition Values (Per Serving)

- Calories: 350
- Fat: 31g
- Carbohydrates: 0.2g
- Protein: 15g

Chicken Scallops

(Prep time: 6 minutes\ Cook time: 8 minutes\ 2 servings)

Ingredients

- 4 boneless, skinless chicken breasts
- 4 Tbsp keto-friendly bread crumbs (or make your own from keto-friendly bread; dry it out, then pulse in food processor to extra-fine consistency)
- 3 Tbsp almond meal
- 2 Tbsp grated parmesan cheese
- 2 Tbsp dried sage
- 2 Tbsp almond flour
- Pinch of salt, pepper
- 2 eggs, beaten
- Garnish: fresh parsley

Directions

1. Rinse the chicken. Pat dry.
2. Place chicken breast between plastic wrap, flatten with a rolling pin to ½ inch thickness.
3. In a medium bowl, combine almond flour, parmesan cheese, and sage. Stir.
4. In a medium bowl, combine bread crumbs, salt, pepper. Stir.
5. In a medium bowl, beat the eggs.
6. Dip chicken breasts in seasoned flour, then egg, then bread crumbs. Place on a tray. Place tray in freezer 5 minutes.
7. Pre-heat the fryer to 390°F. Lightly spray cook basket with non-stick Keto cooking spray.
8. Place breasts in basket; so they aren't touching – may have to cook in batches.
9. Cook chicken breasts 8 minutes; until golden brown and cooked thoroughly.
10. Transfer to serving platter. Garnish with fresh parsley.

Nutrition Values (Per Serving)

- Calories: 272
- Fat: 14g
- Carbohydrates: 14g
- Protein: 20g

Chicken Skewers

(Prep time: 10 minutes\ Cook time: 12 minutes\ 2 servings)

Ingredients

- 4 boneless, skinless chicken thighs
- 1 Tbsp mirin
- 1 tsp garlic salt
- 2½ cups light soy sauce
- 12 pearl onions
- 4 bamboo sticks
- Garnish: fresh green onions, diced

Directions

1. Soak bamboo sticks in water 15 minutes. Rinse the chicken. Pat dry.
2. Cut chicken into bite-size pieces. Clean the onions. Pat dry.
3. Slide on alternating piece of chicken then onion until skewer complete.
4. In a large glass dish, combine the soy sauce, garlic salt, mirin. Stir well.
5. Marinate the skewers in this mixture in refrigerator 2 hours.
6. Pre-heat fryer 350°F. Lightly spray cook basket with non-stick Keto cooking spray.
7. Transfer skewers to your fryer. Cook 12 minutes until cooked thoroughly.
8. Transfer to serving platter. Garnish with green onions.

Nutrition Values (Per Serving)

- Calories: 269
- Fat: 18g
- Carbohydrates: 9g
- Protein: 18g

Country Chicken

(Prep time: 10 minutes\ Cook time: 15 minutes\ 2 servings)

Ingredients

- ¾ pound boneless, skinless fresh chicken tenders
- ½ cup almond meal
- ½ cup almond flour
- 1 tsp dried rosemary
- Pinch of salt, pepper
- 2 eggs, beaten

Directions

1. Rinse the chicken tenders, pat dry.
2. In a medium bowl, pour in almond flour.
3. In a medium bowl, beat the eggs.
4. In a medium bowl, pour in almond meal. Season with rosemary, salt, pepper.
5. Dip chicken pieces in flour, then egg, then almond meal. Set on a tray.
6. Place tray in freezer 5 minutes.
7. Pre-heat fryer to 350°F. Lightly spray cook basket with non-stick Keto cooking spray.
8. Cook tenders 10 minutes. After timer runs out, set temperature to 390°F, cook 5 more minutes until golden brown.
9. Serve on a platter. Side with preferred dipping sauce.

Nutrition Values (Per Serving)

- Calories: 480
- Fat: 36g
- Carbohydrates: 13g
- Protein: 26g

Ginger Chicken Thighs

(Prep time: 5 minutes\ Cook time: 15 minutes\ 2 servings)

Ingredients

- 3 boneless, skinless chicken thighs, diced in bite-size pieces
- 1 shallot, thinly sliced
- ½ cup apple cider
- 1 Tbsp grated ginger
- Pinch of salt, pepper

Directions

1. Rinse chicken with cold water. Pat dry.
2. In a small bowl combine apple cider, ginger, salt, pepper, shallot.
3. Pour into large Ziploc baggie. Add chicken thighs to bag, massage marinade into chicken until evenly coated. Refrigerate 2 hours. When removing from Ziploc, pat dry any excess liquid before cooking.
4. When ready to cook, pre-heat fryer to 350°F. Lightly spray cook basket with non-stick Keto cooking spray.
5. Cook 15 minutes; turn at halfway point.
6. Serve over brown rice or vegetables.

Nutrition Values (Per Serving)

- Calories: 726
- Fat: 48g
- Carbohydrates: 9g
- Protein: 64g

Lime Chicken

(Prep time: 5 minutes\ Cook time: 15 – 20 minutes\ 2 servings)

Ingredients

- 16 chicken wings
- 2 Tbsp light coconut aminos
- 2 Tbsp agave nectar
- 2 Tbsp lemon juice
- Pinch of salt, pepper
- Garnish: sesame seeds

Directions

1. Rinse the chicken thighs. Pat dry.
2. In a large bowl, combine coconut aminos, agave, lemon juice, salt, pepper. Stir.
3. Pour into a Ziploc baggie. Add chicken wings, massage until evenly coated. Refrigerate 2 hours. Remove from fridge, pat dry any excess liquid.
4. Pre-heat fryer to 350°F. Lightly spray cook basket with non-stick Keto cooking spray.
5. Cook 6 minutes, flip and continue cooking 6 more minutes.
6. Flip again. Cook at 390°F 3 more minutes.
7. Serve on a platter. Garnish with sesame seeds.

Nutrition Values (Per Serving)

- Calories: 42
- Fat: 72g
- Carbohydrates: 16g
- Protein: 12g

Schnitzel Parmigiana

(Prep time: 5 minutes\ Cook time: 20 minutes\ 2 servings)

Ingredients

- 1 pre-breaded chicken schnitzel, keto-friendly
- 3 Tbsp pasta sauce, keto-friendly
- ¼ cup grated cheese, your choice

Directions

1. Pre-heat fryer to 350°F. Lightly spray cook basket with non-stick Keto cooking spray.
2. Add schnitzel to the fryer. Cook 15 minutes.
3. Spoon pasta sauce over chicken, top with cheese.
4. Cook 5 minutes until cheese melted.
5. Serve immediately.

Nutrition Values (Per Serving)

- Calories: 190
- Fat: 8g
- Carbohydrates: 5g
- Protein: 13g

Cheesy Chicken Bites

(Prep time: 10 minutes\ Cook time: 8 minutes\ 2 servings)

Ingredients

- 2 x 8 ounce boneless, skinless chicken breasts
- 5 Tbsp almond meal
- 1 Tbsp almond flour
- 2 Tbsp grated parmesan cheese
- 1 tsp garlic salt
- Pinch of pepper
- 1 Tbsp melted butter

Directions

1. Rinse the chicken. Pat dry. Dice into bite-size pieces.
2. In a small bowl, combine almond meal, almond flour, parmesan cheese, garlic salt, pepper. Stir.
3. Melt the butter. Allow to cool slightly.
4. Dip chicken pieces in butter.
5. Dip chicken pieces in almond meal mixture. Place on a tray. Freeze 5 minutes.
6. Pre-heat fryer to 350°F. Lightly spray cook basket with non-stick Keto cooking spray.
7. Place chicken breast pieces in fryer. Cook 6 minutes, flip over, cook 2 more minutes; until cooked thoroughly.
8. Transfer to platter. Garnish with fresh, diced green onion.

Nutrition Values (Per Serving)

- Calories: 266
- Fat: 14g
- Carbohydrates: 16g
- Protein: 12g

Jerk Chicken Wings

(Prep time: 15 minutes\ Cook time: 14 minutes\ 2 servings)

Ingredients

- 1 pound chicken wings (if using boneless, reduce cooking time)
- 1 tsp garlic powder
- ¼ tsp cayenne pepper
- 1 Tbsp prepared mustard
- 1 Tbsp tomato puree
- Pinch of salt, pepper

Directions

1. Rinse chicken wings. Pat dry.
2. In a large bowl, combine the tomato puree, prepared mustard, garlic powder, cayenne pepper, salt, pepper. Stir until combined. Transfer marinade to Ziploc baggie.
3. Add chicken wings. Massage marinade to coat evenly.
4. Allow chicken to marinate 10 minutes.
5. Pre-heat fryer to 350°F. Lightly spray cook basket with non-stick Keto cooking spray.
6. Transfer wings to fryer. Cook 14 minutes; until cooked thoroughly.
7. Transfer to platter.

Nutrition Values (Per Serving)

- Calories: 234
- Fat: 10g
- Carbohydrates: 3g
- Protein: 33g

Chapter 4: Pork, Beef, Lamb

Beef Tongue

(Prep time: 10 minutes\ Cook time: 20 minutes\ 2 servings)

Ingredients

- 1 pound beef tongue
- 1 tsp paprika
- 1 Tbsp butter
- Pinch of salt, pepper

Directions

1. Rinse the beef tongue.
2. Place in a pot with 4 cups of water. Simmer on the stove 30 minutes.
3. Remove from water. Allow to cool slightly. Slice into strips.
4. Melt the butter, allow to cool. Dip the beef tongue strips in butter.
5. Season with paprika, salt, pepper.
6. Pre-heat fryer to 350°F. Lightly spray cook basket with non-stick Keto cooking spray.
7. Transfer beef tongue strips to fryer. Cook 20 minutes.
8. Transfer to platter.

Nutrition Values (Per Serving)

- Calories: 234
- Fat: 18g
- Carbohydrates: 0.4g
- Protein: 14g

Pork Rinds

(Prep time: 10 minutes\ Cook time: 7 minutes\ 2 servings)

Ingredients

- 1 pound pork rinds
- 1 tsp chili flakes
- Pinch of salt, pepper

Directions

1. Pre-heat fryer to 350°F. Lightly spray cook basket with non-stick Keto cooking spray.
2. Place pork rinds, chili flakes, salt, pepper in a Ziploc baggie. Shake until evenly coated.
3. Place in fryer. Cook 7 minutes; shake at halfway cooking point.
4. Transfer to a serving plate.

Nutrition Values (Per Serving)

- Calories: 329
- Fat: 20g
- Carbohydrates: 0.1g
- Protein: 36g

Ribeye Steak

(Prep time: 10 minutes\ Cook time: 13 minutes\ 2 servings)

Ingredients

- 2 pounds ribeye steaks
- Salt and pepper

Directions

1. Pre-heat fryer to 350°F. Lightly spray cook basket with non-stick Keto cooking spray.
2. Bring steaks to room temperature.
3. Season with salt and pepper.
4. Place steaks in the fryer. Cook 7 minutes.
5. Turn the steaks over. Cook another 6 minutes.
6. Serve on a plate. Allow to rest 5 minutes before slicing.

Nutrition Values (Per Serving)

- Calories: 703
- Fat: 58g
- Carbohydrates: 1g
- Protein: 46g

Pork Chops

(Prep time: 10 minutes\ Cook time: 11 minutes\ 3 servings)

Ingredients

- 3 boneless, skinless pork chops
- 1 tsp minced garlic
- ½ tsp rosemary
- 1 Tbsp butter
- Pinch of salt, pepper

Directions

1. Melt the butter. Allow to cool slightly.
2. In a medium bowl, combine the garlic, rosemary, salt, pepper.
3. Dip the pork chops in the butter.
4. Dip the pork chops in the seasoning. Shake off any excess.
5. Pre-heat fryer to 365°F. Lightly spray cook basket with non-stick Keto cooking spray.
6. Place pork chops in the fryer. Cook 6 minutes.
7. Flip, continue cooking 5 more minutes.
8. Serve on a platter.

Nutrition Values (Per Serving)

- Calories: 431
- Fat: 34g
- Carbohydrates: 0.9g
- Protein: 27g

Parmesan Beef

(Prep time: 15 minutes\ Cook time: 20 minutes\ 2 servings)

Ingredients

- 1 pound beef brisket
- 1 tsp dried oregano
- 2 Tbsp italian dressing, keto-friendly
- 2 Tbsp pasta sauce, keto-friendly
- ½ cup shredded parmesan cheese

Directions

1. Slice the brisket into 4 pieces.
2. Pour the italian dressing in a bowl. Stir in the oregano.
3. Dip the pieces in the italian dressing. Shake off any excess.
4. Pre-heat fryer to 365°F. Lightly spray cook basket with non-stick Keto cooking spray.
5. Transfer beef to the fryer. Cook 15 minutes, turn at halfway point.
6. Once cooked, spread pasta sauce over each piece, sprinkle parmesan cheese on top. Cook 5 minutes, until cheese melted.
7. Serve on a platter.

Nutrition Values (Per Serving)

- Calories: 348
- Fat: 18g
- Carbohydrates: 5g
- Protein: 42g

Roast Beef

(Prep time: 15 minutes\ Cook time: 30 minutes\ 2 servings)

Ingredients

- 2 pound lean beef roast
- 1 Tbsp olive oil
- Salt, pepper, and favorite seasoning

Directions

1. Pre-heat fryer to 365°F. Lightly spray cook basket with non-stick Keto cooking spray.
2. Lightly coat the roast with olive oil. Pat dry any excess. Season liberally.
3. Transfer roast to fryer. Cook 20 minutes, flip over, cook 10 more minutes.
4. Transfer to platter. Allow to rest 5 minutes before carving.

Nutrition Values (Per Serving)

- Calories: 170
- Fat: 6g
- Carbohydrates: 2g
- Protein: 29g

Fried Lamb Chops

(Prep time: 5 minutes\ Cook time: 10 minutes\ 2 servings)

Ingredients

- 4 lamb chops
- 1 Tbsp olive oil
- Pinch of salt, pepper
- Garnish: fresh mint leaves

Directions

1. Pre-heat fryer to 350°F. Lightly spray cook basket with non-stick Keto cooking spray.
2. Apply light coat of oil on lamb chops. Season with salt and pepper.
3. Place chops in fryer. Cook 10 minutes; until golden crust forms, interior cooked.
4. Serve on a platter. Garnish with mint leaves.

Nutrition Values (Per Serving)

- Calories: 339
- Carbohydrate: 15g
- Protein: 5g
- Fat: 29g

Pork Roast

(Prep time: 120 minutes\ Cook time: 20 minutes\ 2 servings)

Ingredients

- 2 pounds pork shoulder
- 2 Tbsp liquid stevia
- ⅓ cup coconut aminos
- 1 Tbsp agave nectar
- Pinch of salt, pepper
- Garnish: fresh parsley

Directions

1. Cut the meat into 1-inch pieces.
2. In a bowl, combine liquid stevia, agave nectar, coconut aminos, salt, pepper. Stir well.
3. Place pieces of pork in a deep glass dish. Pour the marinade over the pork. Refrigerate 2 hours. When ready to cook, shake off any excess liquid from pork pieces.
4. Pre-heat fryer to 365°F. Lightly spray cook basket with non-stick Keto cooking spray.
5. Transfer pork to the fryer. Cook 10 minutes; shake after 5 minutes.
6. After 10 minutes cooking, increase temperature to 400°F. Cook 10 more minutes.
7. Transfer to serving dish. Garnish with fresh parsley.

Nutrition Values (Per Serving)

- Calories: 158
- Fat: 14g
- Carbohydrates: 10g
- Protein: 1g

T-Bone

(Prep time: 10 minutes\ Cook time: 8 – 10 minutes\ 2 servings)

Ingredients

- 1½ pound T-bone steak
- ¼ cup dry coffee grains
- 2 Tbsp brown sugar
- 2 Tbsp butter

Directions

1. Melt the butter. Allow to cool.
2. Remove steak from your refrigerator. Bring to room temperature; approx. 30 minutes.
3. In a small bowl, combine coffee grinds, brown sugar. Grind it together.
4. Dip the steak in butter. Season with coffee mixture, shake off any excess.
5. Pre-heat fryer to 400°F. Lightly spray cook basket with non-stick Keto cooking spray.
6. Transfer steak to the fryer. Cook 5 minutes, flip to other side. Cook 3 – 5 more minutes.
7. Once cooked, remove steak. Allow to rest 5 minutes before slicing.

Nutrition Values (Per Serving)

- Calories: 130
- Fat: 5g
- Carbohydrates: 5g
- Protein: 24g

Bacon wrapped Asparagus Spears

(Prep time: 15 minutes\ Cook time: 10 minutes\ 2 servings)

Ingredients

- 20 asparagus spears
- 4 slices bacon
- 1 Tbsp sesame oil
- 1 garlic clove, crushed

Directions

1. In a small bowl, combine the garlic and oil. Stir to combine.
2. Pre-heat fryer to 350°F. Lightly spray cook basket with non-stick Keto cooking spray.
3. Wrap 4 asparagus spears with a slice of bacon.
4. Brush with garlic oil mixture.
5. Place in fryer. Cook 10 minutes.
6. Serve on a platter.

Nutrition Values (Per Serving)

- Calories: 183
- Carbohydrate: 5g
- Protein: 6g
- Fat: 16g

Fried Italian Meatballs

(Prep time: 10 minutes\ Cook time: 10 minutes\ 2 servings)

Ingredients

- ½ pound lean ground beef
- 1 small white onion, minced
- 1 Tbsp fresh parsley, minced
- 1 Tbsp oregano
- 1 egg
- 3 Tbsp almond meal
- Pinch of salt, pepper
- Garnish: diced green onions

Directions

1. In a large bowl, combine ground beef, onion, parsley, oregano, almond meal, egg, salt, pepper. Combine until fully mixed.
2. Roll the meat into bite-size meatballs.
3. Pre-heat fryer to 350°F. Lightly spray cook basket with non-stick Keto cooking spray.
4. Transfer meatballs to fryer. Cook 10 minutes.
5. Transfer to platter. Garnish with diced green onion.

Nutrition Values (Per Serving)

- Calories: 234
- Fat: 18g
- Carbohydrates: 0.4g
- Protein: 14g

Cheese And Ham Pinwheels

(Prep time: 15 minutes\ Cook time: 10 minutes\ 2 servings)

Ingredients

- 1 sheet puff pastry, keto-friendly
- 4 Tbsp gruyere cheese, grated
- 6 – 8 slices ham or prosciutto, diced
- 4 tsp Dijon mustard

Directions

1. Place sheet of pastry on a floured surface.
2. Place ham over pastry. Sprinkle cheese over top.
3. Carefully roll up the pastry from the short edge.
4. Wrap in cling wrap. Refrigerate 30 minutes.
5. Pre-heat fryer to 350°F. Lightly spray cook basket with non-stick Keto cooking spray.
6. Remove rolled pastry from fridge. Slice in ½ inch rounds.
7. Transfer to fryer. Cook 10 minutes until golden brown.
8. Serve on a platter. Side with Dijon mustard.

Nutrition Values (Per Serving)

- Calories: 158
- Fat: 8g
- Carbohydrates: 14g
- Protein: 8g

Bacon Cabbage

(Prep time: 10 minutes\ Cook time: 10 minutes\ 2 servings)

Ingredients

- 4 slices bacon, chopped
- 1 cup white cabbage, shredded
- ½ tsp salt, pepper
- 1 tsp paprika
- 1 tsp butter

Directions

1. Pre-heat fryer to 360°F. Lightly spray cook basket with non-stick Keto cooking spray.
2. Place chopped bacon in the fryer. Cook 5 minutes, until brown.
3. Add butter, cabbage to the fryer. Season with salt, pepper, and paprika. Stir.
4. Cook 5 minutes.
5. Transfer to a serving bowl.

Nutrition Values (Per Serving)

- Calories: 184
- Fat: 13g
- Carbohydrates: 5g
- Protein: 11g

Bacon Brussel Sprouts

(Prep time: 10 minutes\ Cook time: 20 minutes\ 2 servings)

Ingredients

- 6 pieces of bacon, chopped
- 1 pound Brussels sprouts
- 1 Tbsp olive oil
- ½ tsp garlic salt
- Pinch of pepper
- Garnish: crushed walnuts

Directions

1. Chop the bacon.
2. Pre-heat fryer to 360°F. Lightly spray cook basket with non-stick Keto cooking spray.
3. Add chopped bacon to fryer. Cook 5 minutes. Stir well. Cook 5 more minutes.
4. Transfer cooked bacon to a serving bowl.
5. In a medium bowl, lightly season brussel sprouts with oil, garlic salt, pepper.
6. Transfer to fryer. At same temperature, cook 10 minutes. Add bacon to fryer. Stir well.
7. Transfer to platter. Garnish with crushed walnuts.

Nutrition Values (Per Serving)

- Calories: 226
- Fat: 17g
- Carbohydrates: 7g
- Protein: 12g

Chapter 5: Fish And Seafood

Spicy Garlic Shrimp

(Prep time: 20 minutes\ Cook time: 5 minutes\ 2 servings)

Ingredients

- 16 fresh shrimp; shelled, deveined
- 2 Tbsp butter
- 1 tsp each salt, pepper
- 3 garlic cloves, minced
- Garnish: diced green onions, diced

Directions

1. Rinse the shrimp. Pat dry.
2. Melt the butter. Add the garlic, salt, pepper.
3. Dip the shrimp in the butter, shake off excess. Refrigerate 10 minutes.
4. Pre-heat fryer to 325°F. Lightly spray cook basket with non-stick Keto cooking spray.
5. Spray a light layer of oil over the shrimp.
6. Transfer shrimp to fryer. Cook 5 minutes; shake at halfway point.
7. Serve on a platter. Garnish with diced green onions.

Nutrition Values (Per Serving)

- Calories: 127
- Fat: 10g
- Carbohydrates: 3g
- Protein: 7g

Butter And Garlic Salmon

(Prep time: 10 minutes\ Cook time: 10 minutes\ 2 servings)

Ingredients

- 2 salmon fillets
- 3 garlic cloves, minced
- 1 tsp olive oil
- 2 Tbsp butter
- Pinch of salt, pepper
- ½ tsp parsley, basil
- Garnish: fresh dill

Directions

1. Pat dry the salmon fillets. Season the fillets with salt, pepper.
2. Pre-heat fryer to 325°F. Lightly spray cook basket with non-stick Keto cooking spray.
3. Transfer fillets to the fryer. Cook 10 minutes.
4. In a small pot, heat the olive oil. Add minced garlic, parsley, basil. Simmer 5 minutes.
5. Remove from heat. Stir in butter.
6. Plate the salmon fillets, drizzle butter mixture over fillets. Garnish with fresh dill.

Nutrition Values (Per Serving)

- Calories: 440
- Fat: 33g
- Carbohydrates: 6g
- Protein: 29g

Bacon Wrapped Shrimp

(Prep time: 15 minutes\ Cook time: 5 minutes\ 2 servings)

Ingredients

- 16 shrimp; shell removed, deveined
- 8 slices thin sliced bacon; bring to room temperature
- 16 toothpicks
- Garnish: diced green onion

Directions

1. Slice the bacon in half.
2. Wrap half a slice of bacon around piece of shrimp.
3. Slide tooth pick from bottom to top of shrimp.
4. Place shrimp on a tray. Refrigerate 10 minutes.
5. Pre-heat fryer to 375°F. Lightly spray cook basket with non-stick Keto cooking spray.
6. Place shrimp in the fryer. Cook 5 minutes.
7. Transfer to platter. Garnish with diced green onion.

Nutrition Values (Per Serving)

- Calories: 127
- Fat: 10g
- Carbohydrates: 3g
- Protein: 7g

Cajun Shrimp

(Prep time: 10 minutes\ Cook time: 5 minutes\ 2 servings)

Ingredients

- 16 tiger shrimp
- 2 Tbsp corn starch
- 1 tsp each; cayenne pepper, old bay seasoning
- Pinch of salt, pepper
- 1 tsp olive oil

Directions

1. Rinse the shrimp. Pat dry.
2. In a bowl, combine corn starch, cayenne pepper, old bay seasoning, salt, pepper. Stir.
3. In a bowl, add the shrimp. Drizzle olive oil over shrimp to lightly coat.
4. Dip the shrimp in seasoning, shake off any excess.
5. Pre-heat fryer to 375°F. Lightly spray cook basket with non-stick Keto cooking spray.
6. Transfer to fryer. Cook 5 minutes; shake after 2 minutes, until cooked thoroughly.
7. Serve on a platter.

Nutrition Values (Per Serving)

- Calories: 127
- Fat: 10g
- Carbohydrates: 3g
- Protein: 7g

Smoked Trout Frittata

(Prep time: 10 minutes\ Cook time: 15 minutes\ 2 servings)

Ingredients

- 2 smoked trout fillets
- 2 Tbsp olive oil
- 1 small white onion, diced
- 6 Tbsp crème fraiche
- 2 eggs
- ½ Tbsp horseradish
- Pinch of salt, pepper

Directions

1. In a small frying pan, heat the oil. Add diced onion. Sauté 5 minutes. Let it cool down.
2. In a large bowl, beat the eggs. Stir in the cream fraiche, horseradish. Mix well.
3. Dice trout fillets into bite-size pieces. Stir into egg mixture. Season with salt and pepper.
4. Pre-heat fryer to 375°F. Lightly spray cook basket with non-stick Keto cooking spray.
5. Take a pan (cake pan/loaf pan/small dish) that fits in the fryer, grease with butter. Pour the frittata mixture in the pan.
6. Transfer to fryer. Cook 15 minutes; until golden brown.
7. Serve with a side of potatoes, or vegetables.

Nutrition Values (Per Serving)

- Calories: 167
- Fat: 18g
- Carbohydrates: 6g
- Protein: 9g

Pineapple Ham Steak

(Prep time: 10 minutes\ Cook time: 10 minutes\ 2 servings)

Ingredients

- 2 large ham steaks
- 4 pieces pineapple, in natural juice
- 1 tsp pineapple juice
- 1 tsp dark brown sugar
- Garnish: fresh mint

Directions

1. In a bowl, combine brown sugar, pineapple juice. Stir well.
2. Slice the ham in half. Rub the brown sugar mixture on both sides.
3. Pre-heat fryer to 350°F. Lightly spray cook basket with non-stick Keto cooking spray.
4. Transfer to fryer. Cook 10 minutes, flip at 5 minute mark.
5. Serve on a platter. Garnish with fresh mint.

Nutrition Values (Per Serving)

- Calories: 258
- Fat: 8g
- Carbohydrates: 17g
- Protein: 24g

Fried Cod

(Prep time: 10 minutes\ Cook time: 10 minutes\ 2 servings)

Ingredients

- 4 cod fillets
- 1 Tbsp olive oil
- Pinch of salt, pepper
- Garnish: fresh basil, fresh lemon slices

Directions

1. Rinse the cod. Lightly coat with olive oil. Season with salt, pepper.
2. Pre-heat fryer to 350°F. Lightly spray cook basket with non-stick Keto cooking spray. Transfer fillets to fryer. Cook 10 minutes, turn at hallway mark.
3. Serve on a platter over brown rice, mixed vegetables.

Nutrition Values (Per Serving)

- Calories: 107
- Fat: 7g
- Carbohydrates: 3g
- Protein: 4g

Crab Sticks

(Prep time: 5 minutes\ Cook time: 15 minutes\ 2 servings)

Ingredients

- 1 pack of DODO or similar crabsticks
- 2 tsp sesame oil
- Dash of curry or cajun seasoning

Directions

1. Dice the crab sticks into bite-size pieces.
2. Place pieces in a bowl. Drizzle light layer sesame oil over crab pieces, toss to evenly coat. Season with curry or cajun seasoning.
3. Pre-heat fryer to 375°F. Lightly spray cook basket with non-stick Keto cooking spray. Transfer to the fryer. Cook 15 minutes; shake at halfway point.
4. Transfer to platter. Garnish with lemon wedges, cocktail sauce.

Nutrition Values (Per Serving)

- Calories: 125
- Fat: 12g
- Carbohydrates: 3g
- Protein: 5g

Fish Nuggets

(Prep time: 5 minutes\ Cook time: 10 minutes\ 2 servings)

Ingredients

- ½ pound fresh fish fillets; choose a mix of cod, sole, halibut
- 2 Tbsp olive oil
- ½ cup almond flour
- 2 large eggs
- 1½ cups almond meal
- Pinch of salt, pepper, fresh thyme
- Garnish: fresh thyme, lemon slices

Directions

1. Rinse the fillets. Pat dry. Dice into bite-size cubes. Lightly coat with olive oil.
2. Pour the almond flour in a bowl. Beat the eggs in a separate bowl.
3. Combine almond meal, salt, pepper, thyme. Mix together.
4. Dip fish pieces in flour, then egg, then seasoned almond meal. Place in a single layer on a tray. Place tray in freezer for 5 minutes.
5. Pre-heat fryer to 375°F. Lightly spray cook basket with non-stick Keto cooking spray.
6. Place fish nuggets in the fryer. Cook 10 minutes, flip at halfway point.
7. Transfer to serving platter. Garnish with fresh thyme, lemon slices.

Nutrition Values (Per Serving)

- Calories: 242
- Fat: 15g
- Carbohydrates: 11g
- Protein: 16g

Squid Rings

(Prep time: 5 minutes\ Cook time: 15 minutes\ 2 servings)

Ingredients

- 12 small rings frozen squid
- 1 large egg
- 1 cup almond flour
- 1 tsp coriander seeds, ground
- Pinch of salt, pepper
- 1 tsp cayenne pepper
- Garnish: lemon slices

Directions

1. In a large bowl, combine flour, coriander seeds, cayenne pepper, salt, pepper. Mix.
2. Coat squid rings with egg mixture then flour. Shake off any excess. Place on a tray. Set in the freezer for 5 minutes.
3. Cover bottom of fryer with parchment paper. Lightly spray parchment with oil.
4. Pre-heat fryer to 375°F. Place squid rings in the fryer.
5. Spray the squid rings with oil Cook 15 minutes; flip over at halfway point, spray with more oil. Continue cooking until golden brown.
6. Transfer to plater. Garnish with lemon slices, and tartar sauce.

Nutrition Values (Per Serving)

- Calories: 227
- Fat: 14g
- Carbohydrates: 14g
- Protein: 11g

Almond Crusted Halibut

(Prep time: 10 minutes\ Cook time: 15 minutes\ 2 servings)

Ingredients

- 4 halibut fillets
- 2 Tbsp sesame oil
- 2 Tbsp almond flour
- 1 cups almond meal
- 1 tsp fresh lemon zest
- Pinch of salt, pepper
- 1 egg
- Garnish: fresh dill, lemon slices

Directions

1. Rinse the fillets. Pat dry.
2. In a bowl, combine almond meal, fresh lemon zest. Stir.
3. In a bowl, beat the egg.
4. Dip fish in fillets in flour, then egg, then almond meal. Place on a tray. Set the tray in freezer 5 minutes.
5. Pre-heat fryer to 350°F. Lightly spray cook basket with non-stick Keto cooking spray.
6. Place fish in the fryer. Cook 15 minutes; flip over at halfway point.
7. Transfer to platter. Garnish with fresh dill, lemon slices.

Nutrition Values (Per Serving)

- Calories: 385
- Fat: 24g
- Carbohydrates: 14g
- Protein: 32g

Catfish

(Prep time: 10 minutes\ Cook time: 20 minutes\ 2 servings)

Ingredients

- 4 pieces of catfish fillets
- ¼ cup seasoning (combination: pinch of dill weed, basil, onion powder, garlic powder, celery seed, oregano, lemon zest, fresh ground black pepper)
- 1 Tbsp olive oil
- Garnish: fresh parsley, lemon slices, tartar sauce

Directions

1. Rinse the catfish. Pat dry.
2. Add fish seasoning to large Ziploc baggie.
3. Lightly coat catfish with olive oil. Place fish in baggie, toss until evenly coated.
4. Pre-heat fryer to 350°F. Lightly spray cook basket with non-stick Keto cooking spray.
5. Transfer fillets to the fryer. Cook 10 minutes, flip over, cook 10 more minutes.
6. Serve on a platter. Garnish with fresh parsley, lemon slices, tartar sauce.

Nutrition Values (Per Serving)

- Calories: 199
- Fat: 12g
- Carbohydrates: 14g
- Protein: 16g

Chapter 6: Vegan And Vegetarian

Buffalo Cauliflower

(Prep time: 20 minutes\ Cook time: 15 minutes\ 2 servings)

Ingredients

- 4 cups cauliflower florets
- 1 cup almond meal
- ¼ cup melted butter
- ¼ cup buffalo sauce

Directions

1. Melt butter. Add buffalo sauce. Stir well.
2. Place florets in a large Ziploc baggie. Pour in marinade. Toss to evenly coat.
3. Roll the florets in almond meal. Shake off any excess. Place on a tray.
4. Set the tray in the freezer for 5 minutes.
5. Pre-heat fryer to 350°F. Lightly spray cook basket with non-stick Keto cooking spray.
6. Transfer florets to the fryer. Cook 15 minutes; shake at halfway point.
7. Serve on a platter. Side with Keto friendly dipping sauce.

Nutrition Values (Per Serving)

- Calories: 382
- Fat: 30g
- Carbohydrates: 18g
- Protein: 5g

Apple Chips

(Prep time: 10 minutes\ Cook time: 10 minutes\ 2 servings)

Ingredients

- 4 red apples
- 1 Tbsp sesame oil
- 1 tsp keto-friendly granulated sugar
- Pinch of ground cinnamon

Directions

1. Core the apples. Leave the peel on. Slice the apples in thin, round circles.
2. Place slices in a large Ziploc baggie. Pour in sesame oil. Massage to coat.
3. Combine granulated sugar, cinnamon in a bowl. Stir.
4. Pour in with apples. Shake to coat evenly.
5. Pre-heat fryer to 325°F. Lightly spray cook basket with non-stick Keto cooking spray.
6. Transfer to the fryer. Cook 10 minutes; shake at halfway point.
7. Serve on a platter. Allow to cool before eating.

Nutrition Values (Per Serving)

- Calories: 22
- Fat: 2g
- Carbohydrates: 5g
- Protein: 0g

Fried Dill Pickles

(Prep time: 15 minutes\ Cook time: 10 minutes\ 2 servings)

Ingredients

- 6 large dill pickles
- 2 eggs
- 2 Tbsp almond flour
- ⅔ cup almond meal
- ⅓ cup finely grated parmesan cheese
- ¼ tsp dried dill weed

Directions

1. Slice the pickles in circles, about ¼ inch thick. Dry with paper towel.
2. Pour almond flour in a bowl. Crack eggs in a bowl, beat well.
3. In a bowl, combine almond meal, dill weed. Mix together.
4. Dip pickles in almond flour, then egg, then almond meal, shake off any excess.
5. Place on a tray. Set tray in freezer 5 minutes.
6. Pre-heat fryer to 350°F. Lightly spray cook basket with non-stick Keto cooking spray.
7. Transfer pickles to the fryer. Cook 10 minutes; shake at halfway point.
8. Transfer to a platter. Serve with Keto-friendly dipping sauce.

Nutrition Values (Per Serving)

- Calories: 94
- Fat: 2g
- Carbohydrates: 12g
- Protein: 3g

Avocado Fries

(Prep time: 20 minutes\ Cook time: 10 minutes\ 2 servings)

Ingredients

- ½ cup almond meal
- ½ tsp salt
- 1 avocado peeled, pitted and cut into ¼ inch fries
- Aquafaba, for coating

Directions

1. Peel the avocado, remove the pit, slice in fries.
2. Take a bowl and mix almond meal and salt.
3. Take another bowl and add aquafaba.
4. Dip the avocado slices in aquafaba and roll in almond meal.
5. Pre-heat fryer to 350°F. Lightly spray cook basket with non-stick Keto cooking spray.
6. Place avocado fries in the fryer. Cook 10 minutes; shake at halfway point.
7. Transfer to a platter. Serve with Keto-friendly dipping sauce.

Nutrition Values (Per Serving)

- Calories: 242
- Fat: 20g
- Carbohydrates: 14g
- Protein: 4g

Fried Brussel Sprouts

(Prep time: 20 minutes\ Cook time: 15 minutes\ 2 servings)

Ingredients

- 1 cup Brussel sprouts
- 1 Tbsp olive oil
- Pinch of salt, pepper
- Garnish: pine nuts

Directions

1. Trim ends off the brussel sprouts. Add to a pot of boiling water. Boil 4 minutes.
2. Transfer to cold water. Drain. Pat dry.
3. Coat lightly in olive oil. Season with salt, pepper.
4. Pre-heat fryer to 350°F. Lightly spray cook basket with non-stick Keto cooking spray.
5. Transfer to the fryer. Cook 15 minutes; shake at halfway point.
6. Serve on a platter. Garnish with pine nuts.

Nutrition Values (Per Serving)

- Calories: 115
- Fat: 4g
- Carbohydrates: 13g
- Protein: 9g

Winter Veggies

(Prep time: 20 minutes\ Cook time: 20 minutes\ 2 servings)

Ingredients

- 1cup diced parsnips
- 1cup diced celery
- 1 small red onion, diced
- 1cup diced butternut squash
- 2 Tbsp olive oil
- Pinch of salt and pepper
- Garnish: fresh dill

Directions

1. Place diced vegetables in a large Ziploc baggie.
2. Lightly coat with olive oil. Season with salt and pepper.
3. Pre-heat fryer to 350°F. Lightly spray cook basket with non-stick Keto cooking spray.
4. Place in the fryer. Cook 20 minutes; shake at the halfway point.
5. Transfer to serving platter. Garnish with fresh dill.

Nutrition Values (Per Serving)

- Calories: 382
- Fat: 30g
- Carbohydrates: 18g
- Protein: 5g

Roasted Carrots

(Prep time: 10 minutes\ Cook time: 20 minutes\ 2 servings)

Ingredients

- 10 small carrots
- 1 Tbsp olive oil
- 1 tsp cumin seeds
- Garnish: fresh coriander

Directions

1. Peel and dice the carrots. Rinse. Pat dry.
2. Lightly coat carrots with olive oil. Grind up the cumin seeds.
3. Season the carrots with cumin.
4. Pre-heat fryer to 350°F. Lightly spray cook basket with non-stick Keto cooking spray. Place carrots in the fryer. Cook 20 minutes; shake at halfway point.
5. Transfer to platter. Garnish with fresh coriander.

Nutrition Values (Per Serving)

- Calories: 131
- Fat: 7g
- Carbohydrates: 15g
- Protein: 2g

Banana Chips

(Prep time: 10 minutes\ Cook time: 15 minutes\ 2 servings)

Ingredients

- 3 bananas
- ½ tsp turmeric powder
- ½ tsp Chat masala
- 1 Tbsp flavorless oil

Directions

1. Peel and slice the bananas to ¼ inch thickness.
2. In a bowl, combine turmeric, masala.
3. Place the banana pieces in a large Ziploc. Lightly coat with oil. Add the seasoning. Massage until evenly coated.
4. Pre-heat fryer to 350°F. Lightly spray cook basket with non-stick Keto cooking spray. Place in the fryer. Cook 15 minutes; shake at halfway point.
5. Transfer to bowl. Cool before eating.

Garlic Green Peppers

(Prep time: 10 minutes\ Cook time: 15 minutes\ 2 servings)

Ingredients

- 1 pound green peppers
- 1 tsp minced garlic
- 1 tsp salt, pepper
- 1 Tbsp olive oil
- Garnish: fresh parsley

Directions

1. Wash the green peppers, deseed. Slice in strips. Pat dry.
2. Place in a Ziploc baggie. Drizzle oil over the pieces.
3. Add the garlic, salt, pepper. Massage to coat lightly.
4. Pre-heat fryer to 325°F. Lightly spray cook basket with non-stick Keto cooking spray.
5. Place in the fryer. Cook 15 minutes; shake at halfway point.
6. Transfer to platter. Garnish with fresh parsley.

Nutrition Values (Per Serving)

- Calories: 54
- Fat: 0.6g
- Carbohydrates: 5g
- Protein: 1g

Curried Cauliflower

(Prep time: 15 minutes\ Cook time: 15 minutes\ 2 servings)

Ingredients

- 1 small head of cauliflower
- 1 tsp curry powder
- 4 tsp olive oil
- 1 tsp salt

Directions

1. Peel off the leaves. Dice the cauliflower into bite-size pieces.
2. Place the florets in a Ziploc baggie. Drizzle light layer of oil over the florets.
3. Shake in curry powder and salt. Massage the florets until evenly coated.
4. Pre-heat fryer to 350°F. Lightly spray cook basket with non-stick Keto cooking spray.
5. Place florets in the fryer. Cook 15 minutes; shake at halfway point.
6. Transfer to serving platter. Side with Keto-friendly dipping sauce.

Stuffed Peppers

(Prep time: 20 minutes\ Cook time: 10 minutes\ 2 servings)

Ingredients

- 8 mini bell peppers
- 1 tsp black pepper
- ½ Tbsp of Italian herbs
- ½ Tbsp olive oil
- ¼ cup goat cheese, softened
- Garnish: fresh parsley

Directions

1. Slice the tops off the mini peppers, remove the seeds.
2. Wipe with a damp cloth.
3. In a bowl, combine italian herbs, black pepper with goat cheese. Stir until smooth.
4. Stuff the peppers with goat cheese mixture. Lightly coat the mini peppers with the oil.
5. Pre-heat fryer to 350°F. Lightly spray cook basket with non-stick Keto cooking spray.
6. Place mini peppers in the fryer. Cook 10 minutes; until peppers are tender.
7. Transfer to a platter. Garnish with fresh parsley.

Nutrition Values (Per Serving)

- Calories: 122
- Fat: 2g
- Carbohydrates: 14g
- Protein: 9g

Fried Pumpkin Seeds

(Prep time: 10 minutes\ Cook time: 20 minutes\ 2 servings)

Ingredients

- 1½ cups pumpkin seeds
- 1 tsp flavorless oil
- 1½ tsp salt
- 1 tsp smoked paprika

Directions

1. Cut open the pumpkin, Scrape out the seeds.
2. Rinse them under cool water until clean. Dry them well.
3. Place the pumpkin seeds in a Ziploc baggie. Lightly coat with flavorless oil.
4. Add the salt and smoked paprika to the baggie. Massage through the bag to coat evenly.
5. Pre-heat fryer to 350°F. Lightly spray cook basket with non-stick Keto cooking spray.
6. Place the pumpkin seeds in the fryer. Cook 20 minutes; shake at halfway point.
7. Transfer to a bowl. Cool completely before eating.

Nutrition Values (Per Serving)

- Calories: 184
- Fat: 16g
- Carbohydrates: 4g
- Protein: 16g

Fried Parsnips

(Prep time: 15 minutes\ Cook time: 15 minutes\ 2 servings)

Ingredients

- 3 parsnips
- 2 Tbsp almond flour
- Pinch of ginger, ground cinnamon
- 2 Tbsp flavorless oil
- Dash of salt

Directions

1. Peel the parsnip. Slice like french fries. Rinse and pat dry.
2. Place parsnip slices in a Ziploc baggie.
3. Add the oil. Massage through bag to coat evenly.
4. In a bowl combine flour, ginger, ground cinnamon, salt. Sprinkle over parsnips to coat.
5. Pre-heat fryer to 350°F. Lightly spray cook basket with non-stick Keto cooking spray.
6. Place parsnips in the fryer. Cook 15 minutes; shake at halfway point.
7. Transfer to a serving bowl.

Nutrition Values (Per Serving)

- Calories: 228
- Fat: 17g
- Carbohydrates: 15g
- Protein: 17g

Kale Chips

(Prep time: 5 minutes\ Cook time: 5 minutes\ 2 servings)

Ingredients

- 4 cups kale
- 2 Tbsp olive oil
- 2 tsp vegan ranch seasoning
- 1 Tbsp nutritional yeast
- ¼ tsp salt

Directions

1. Rinse the kale. Dry thoroughly.
2. In a small bowl, combine the oil, ranch dressing, yeast, salt. Stir well.
3. Place the kale in a large Ziploc baggie. Drizzle in the oil for a light coating.
4. Shake in seasoning mixture. Massage through the bag to coat evenly.
5. Pre-heat fryer to 375°F. Lightly spray cook basket with non-stick Keto cooking spray.
6. Place the kale in the fryer. Cook 5 minutes; shake at halfway point.
7. Transfer to serving platter. Cool completely before eating.

Nutrition Values (Per Serving)

- Calories: 110
- Fat: 5g
- Carbohydrates: 16g
- Protein: 76g

Spicy Asparagus

(Prep time: 15 minutes\ Cook time: 10 minutes\ 2 servings)

Ingredients

- 1 pound asparagus
- 1 tsp salt, white pepper
- 1 tsp chili flakes
- 1 Tbsp flax seeds
- 1 Tbsp sesame oil

Directions

1. Wipe the asparagus with a damp cloth. Cut off woodsy end.
2. In a bowl, combine the salt, pepper, chili flakes, flax seed. Grind together.
3. Lightly coat the asparagus with sesame oil. Season with mixture.
4. Pre-heat fryer to 350°F. Lightly spray cook basket with non-stick Keto cooking spray.
5. Place asparagus in the fryer. Cook 10 minutes; turn at halfway point.
6. Transfer to platter.

Nutrition Values (Per Serving)

- Calories: 42
- Fat: 2g
- Carbohydrates: 3g
- Protein: 1g

Zucchini Gratin

(Prep time: 15 minutes\ Cook time: 15 minutes\ 2 servings)

Ingredients

- 2 whole zucchini
- 1 Tbsp coconut flour
- ¼ cup finely shredded parmesan cheese
- 1 tsp butter
- Pinch of salt, pepper
- Garnish: fresh parsley

Directions

1. Wipe the zucchini with a damp cloth. Don't peel. Slice in ½ inch circles.
2. Melt the butter. Allow to cool slightly.
3. In a bowl, combine coconut flour, shredded cheese, salt, pepper.
4. Place sliced zucchini in a large Ziploc baggie. Drizzle in butter.
5. Sprinkle flour/cheese mixture over zucchini. Massage to coat evenly.
6. Pre-heat fryer to 400°F. Lightly spray cook basket with non-stick Keto cooking spray.
7. Place zucchini in the fryer. Cook 15 minutes; shake at halfway point.
8. Transfer to platter. Garnish with fresh parsley.

Nutrition Values (Per Serving)

- Calories: 98
- Fat: 6g
- Carbohydrates: 5g
- Protein: 10g

Spaghetti Squash

(Prep time: 15 minutes\ Cook time: 30 minutes\ 2 servings)

Ingredients

- 1 medium winter squash
- 2 Tbsp dried chicken stock
- Pinch of black pepper
- 1 cup mixed vegetables; cherry tomatoes, sweet peppers
- 1 tsp butter

Directions

1. Wipe the squash, tomatoes, sweet peppers with a damp cloth.
2. Set the tomatoes, peppers aside. Slice the squash in half.
3. Drizzle oil over inside of squash halves. Season with salt, pepper.
4. Pre-heat fryer to 375°F. Lightly spray cook basket with non-stick Keto cooking spray.
5. Place squash halves in the fryer. Cook 20 minutes.
6. In a bowl, combine dried chicken stock, tomatoes, sweet peppers.
7. Open the fryer. Set the vegetables in shell of squash halves. Cook another 10 minutes.
8. Remove squash from fryer. Remove vegetables from the squash. Set in a bowl.
9. Scrape out the squash with a fork. Serve in a bowl. Top with cooked vegetables.

Nutrition Values (Per Serving)

- Calories: 55
- Fat: 3g
- Carbohydrates: 5g
- Protein: 0.7g

Cabbage Steaks

(Prep time: 10 minutes\ Cook time: 10 minutes\ 2 servings)

Ingredients

- 1 small head of cabbage
- 1 tsp salt, black pepper
- 1 tsp butter
- 1 tsp paprika
- 1 tsp olive oil

Directions

1. Peel off outer tough layers of cabbage. Wipe with a damp cloth.
2. Melt butter. Combine with oil.
3. Slice cabbage in large circles ½ inch thick.
4. Place sliced cabbage on a tray. Drizzle light layer of oil on both sides of cabbage.
5. Season with paprika, salt, pepper.
6. Pre-heat fryer to 375°F. Lightly spray cook basket with non-stick Keto cooking spray.
7. Place cabbage in the fryer. Cook 10 minutes; turn after 5 minutes.
8. Transfer to platter.

Nutrition Values (Per Serving)

- Calories: 37
- Fat: 3g
- Carbohydrates: 5g
- Protein: 0.9g

Eggplant Parmesan

(Prep time: 10 minutes\ Cook time: 15 minutes\ 2 servings)

Ingredients

- 1 large eggplant
- 1 Tbsp canola oil
- ½ tsp chili powder
- 1 tsp garlic powder
- Pinch of salt, pepper
- ¼ cup shredded parmesan cheese

Directions

1. Wipe down eggplant with damp cloth.
2. Slice in circles ½ inch thick. Place in a large Ziploc baggie.
3. Drizzle oil over eggplant. Massage to coat evenly.
4. In a bowl, combine chili powder, garlic powder, salt, pepper.
5. Pre-heat fryer to 400°F. Lightly spray cook basket with non-stick Keto cooking spray.
6. Place slices in the fryer. Cook 15 minutes.
7. Sprinkle parmesan cheese over each slice. Cook 2 more minutes until melted.
8. Transfer to a platter.

Nutrition Values (Per Serving)

- Calories: 115
- Fat: 9g
- Carbohydrates: 3g
- Protein: 7g

Green and Yellow Beans

(Prep time: 10 minutes\ Cook time: 10 minutes\ 2 servings)

Ingredients

- ½ pound green and yellow beans
- 1 Tbsp almond meal
- 1 Tbsp butter
- 1 Tbsp olive oil
- 1 Tbsp combined; parsley, thyme, basil
- Pinch salt, ground white pepper
- Garnish: fresh herbs

Directions

1. Trim ends of beans. Wipe with damp cloth.
2. In a medium bowl, melt the butter. Stir in the oil.
3. In a bowl, combine the almond meal, herbs, salt, pepper.
4. Transfer beans to Ziploc bag. Drizzle in butter mixture. Season with herb mixture.
5. Massage through bag to coat evenly. Shake off any excess as you place them in the fryer.
6. Pre-heat fryer to 325°F. Lightly spray cook basket with non-stick Keto cooking spray.
7. Cook 10 minutes; shake at halfway point.
8. Transfer to a platter. Garnish with more fresh herbs.

Nutrition Values (Per Serving)

- Calories: 90
- Fat: 6g
- Carbohydrates: 8g
- Protein: 2g

Tofu

(Prep time: 10 minutes\ Cook time: 20 minutes\ 2 servings)

Ingredients

- ½ pound tofu
- ½ tsp low sodium soy sauce
- 1 Tbsp almond meal
- 1 tsp onion powder
- 1 tsp garlic powder
- 1 tsp chili flakes
- ¼ cup finely shredded parmesan cheese
- 1 tsp salt, pepper
- Garnish: fresh parsley

Directions

1. Strain the tofu; remove all moisture. Dice into ½ inch chunks. Transfer to a bowl.
2. Drizzle a light layer of soy sauce over the pieces.
3. In a bowl, combine almond meal, onion powder, garlic powder, chili flakes, salt, pepper.
4. Coat the tofu pieces with the mixture. Remove any excess.
5. Pre-heat fryer to 375°F. Lightly spray cook basket with non-stick Keto cooking spray.
6. Transfer pieces to the fryer. Cook 20 minutes; shaking at halfway point.
7. Transfer to platter. Garnish with fresh parsley.

Nutrition Values (Per Serving)

- Calories: 76
- Fat: 4.8g
- Carbohydrates: 1.9g
- Protein: 8g

Zucchini Zoodles

(Prep time: 15 minutes\ Cook time: 5 minutes\ 2 servings)

Ingredients

- 1 whole zucchini
- ¼ cup vegetable stock
- Pinch of salt, pepper
- Garnish: fresh parmesan cheese, fresh parsley

Directions

1. Peel the zucchini. Pass through a Spiralizer.
2. Pre-heat fryer to 375°F. Lightly spray cook basket with non-stick Keto cooking spray.
3. Pour stock in the fryer. Cook 2 minutes. Add the zoodles. Season with salt and pepper.
4. Cook 3 more minutes.
5. Transfer to platter. Top with shredded parmesan cheese, fresh parsley.

Nutrition Values (Per Serving)

- Calories: 19
- Fat: 2g
- Carbohydrates: 2g
- Protein: 0.8g

Onion Rings

(Prep time: 15 minutes\ Cook time: 10 minutes\ 2 servings)

Ingredients

- 1 large yellow onion
- ¼ cup almond flour
- 2 Tbsp almond milk, or any other milk choice
- ¼ cup almond meal
- ¼ tsp salt
- ¼ tsp paprika

Directions

1. Peel the onion. Slice to ½ inch thickness. Separate the onion pieces.
2. Combine the almond flour, and almond milk. Stir well.
3. Combine the bread crumbs with salt, paprika. Mix well.
4. Dip the onion pieces in liquid mixture then the bread crumbs. Place on a tray.
5. Set tray in the freezer 5 minutes.
6. Pre-heat fryer to 390°F. Lightly spray cook basket with non-stick Keto cooking spray.
7. Place onions in the fryer. Cook 10 minutes; flip at halfway point.
8. Transfer to platter. Side with Keto-friendly dressing.

Nutrition Values (Per Serving)

- Calories: 98
- Fat: 1g
- Carbohydrates: 14g
- Protein: 4g

Turnips

(Prep time: 10 minutes\ Cook time: 15 minutes\ 2 servings)

Ingredients

- 5 whole turnips
- ½ white onion, sliced
- 1 Tbsp butter
- 1 tsp salt
- 1 Tbsp almond meal

Directions

1. Peel the turnips and slice to ¼ inch thickness. Wipe with damp cloth.
2. Melt the butter. Place the turnip pieces in a bowl. Pour the butter over top.
3. In a bowl, combine the almond meal and salt. Dip the turnip pieces in almond meal. Place on a tray. Set tray in freezer for 5 minutes.
4. Pre-heat fryer to 400°F. Lightly spray cook basket with non-stick Keto cooking spray.
5. Don't add a coating to the onions. Place turnip pieces and diced onion in the fryer. Cook 15 minutes; shake at halfway point.
6. Transfer to a platter. Season with salt if needed.

Nutrition Values (Per Serving)

- Calories: 206
- Fat: 19g
- Carbohydrates: 8g
- Protein: 2g

Radish Chips

(Prep time: 8 minutes\ Cook time: 15 minutes\ 2 servings)

Ingredients

- 10 radishes
- 2 Tbsp olive oil
- 1 tsp salt

Directions

1. Wash the radishes. Pat dry. Slice into chip slices
2. Drizzle a light layer of olive oil over sliced radishes. Season with salt.
3. Pre-heat fryer to 375°F. Lightly spray cook basket with non-stick Keto cooking spray.
4. Place radish slices in the fryer. Cook 15 minutes; shake at halfway point.
5. Transfer to platter. Allow to cool slightly before eating.

Nutrition Values (Per Serving)

- Calories: 26
- Fat: 3g
- Carbohydrates: 1.3g
- Protein: 0.3g

Chapter 7: Appetizers

Bread

(Prep time: 20 minutes\ Cook time: 30 minutes\ 2 servings)

Ingredients

- 1 cup almond flour
- 3 eggs
- ¼ cup butter
- 1 tsp baking powder
- ¼ tsp salt

Directions

1. Melt the butter. Allow to cool to room temperature.
2. In a small bowl, beat the eggs. Add butter to eggs.
3. In a separate bowl, combine almond flour, salt, baking powder. Mix.
4. Add the dry to the wet. Stir slowly until the mixture comes away from the sides of the bowl. Pour out onto floured surface. Knead the dough until smooth; a few minutes. Lightly grease a glass bowl. Place dough in bowl. Cover with towel. Allow to rest 10 minutes. Shape into a loaf. Do not spray baking dish. Transfer dough to baking dish.
5. Pre-heat fryer to 390°F. Transfer pan to the fryer. Cook 15 minutes.
6. Reduce temperature to 350°F. Cook 15 more minutes.
7. Transfer bread to wooden board. Allow to cool before slicing.

Nutrition Values (Per Serving)

- Calories: 40
- Fat: 3.9g
- Carbohydrates: 0.5g
- Protein: 1.2g

Scrambled Eggs

(Prep time: 10 minutes\ Cook time: 4 minutes\ 2 servings)

Ingredients

- 3 Tbsp milk
- 1 tsp butter
- 3 eggs
- Pinch of salt, pepper

Directions

1. In a bowl, combine the eggs with milk, salt, pepper. Whisk briskly.
2. Lightly grease an air fryer safe dish with butter. Pour egg mixture in dish.
3. Pre-heat fryer to 375°F. Transfer dish to the fryer. Bake 4 minutes.
4. Remove from the fryer. Serve with brown toast.

Nutrition Values (Per Serving)

- Calories: 468
- Fat: 32g
- Carbohydrates: 2g
- Protein: 42g

Egg Soufflé

(Prep time: 10 minutes\ Cook time: 8 minutes\ 2 servings)

Ingredients

- 4 eggs
- 4 Tbsp light cream
- 1 small red chili pepper, diced small
- Few leaves fresh parsley, chopped

Directions

1. In a bowl, combine eggs, cream, red chili pepper, parsley. Stir until combined.
2. Divide mixture evenly between soufflé dishes; filling ½ way. (Do not grease dishes.)
3. Pre-heat fryer to 390°F. Place in the fryer. Cook 8 minutes.
4. Serve with a side of cooked vegetables.

Nutrition Values (Per Serving)

- Calories: 407
- Fat: 23g
- Carbohydrates: 4g
- Protein: 45g

Cheesy Sweet Potatoes

(Prep time: 15 minutes\ Cook time: 25 minutes\ 2 servings)

Ingredients

- 4 small sweet potatoes
- 2 Tbsp butter
- ½ cup finely shredded mozzarella cheese
- Pinch of salt, pepper
- Garnish: diced fresh chives

Directions

1. Scrub and dry the potatoes. Poke holes in the skin (allows steam to release).
2. You could run potatoes 5 minutes in microwave to give them a cooking head start.
3. Pre-heat fryer to 375°F. Lightly spray cook basket with non-stick Keto cooking spray.
4. Place potatoes in the fryer. Cook 25 minutes; turn at halfway point.
5. Once cooked, remove potatoes from fryer. Split open, scoop out filling.
6. Place filling in bowl. Add butter, salt, pepper. Return filling to potatoes.
7. Return potatoes to the fryer. Sprinkle shredded cheese on top. Cook until cheese melts.
8. Transfer potatoes to platter. Garnish with fresh chives.

Nutrition Values (Per Serving)

- Calories: 293
- Fat: 18g
- Carbohydrates: 15g
- Protein: 16g

Vegetable Parmesan Bites

(Prep time: 8 minutes\ Cook time: 10 minutes\ 2 servings)

Ingredients

- 1 small zucchini
- 1 small yellow squash
- 1 small white potatoe
- 1 small tomato
- 1 Tbsp olive oil
- ½ tsp turmeric
- ½ tsp garlic powder
- ¼ tsp salt, white pepper
- ½ cup finely shredded mozzarella cheese
- 2 Tbsp finely shredded parmesan cheese
- Garnish: fresh parsley, fresh ground black pepper

Directions

1. Wipe all the vegetables with a damp cloth. Slice the vegetables ¼ inch thick.
2. Place them all in a baggie. Lightly drizzle olive oil into bag, massage to coat evenly.
3. Season with turmeric, salt, pepper.
4. Pre-heat fryer to 375°F. Lightly spray cook basket with non-stick Keto cooking spray.
5. Place vegetables in the fryer. Cook 10 minutes; turn at halfway point.
6. Combine mozzarella and parmesan cheese together.
7. Once vegetables cooked, sprinkle cheese over top. Cook until melted (couple minutes).
8. Transfer to platter. Garnish with fresh parsley, fresh ground black pepper.

Nutrition Values (Per Serving)

- Calories: 131
- Fat: 8g
- Carbohydrates: 8g
- Protein: 10g

Carrot Fries

(Prep time: 10 minutes\ Cook time: 15 minutes\ 2 servings)

Ingredients

- 10 medium carrots
- 1 Tbsp flavorless oil
- 1 Tbsp almond meal
- 1 tsp dried dill
- Pinch of salt, pepper
- Garnish: fresh dill, keto-friendly ranch dressing

Directions

1. Scrub the carrots, don't peel them. Pat dry.
2. Dice into french fries (not too thick).
3. Place carrots in a large Ziploc baggie. Drizzle in light layer of oil.
4. In a bowl, combine almond meal with salt, pepper. Dip carrots in almond meal, shake off excess. Place on a tray. Set tray in freezer for 5 minutes.
5. Pre-heat fryer to 375°F. Lightly spray cook basket with non-stick Keto cooking spray.
6. Place carrot sticks in the fryer. Cook 15 minutes; shake at halfway point.
7. Transfer to platter. Garnish with fresh dill. Serve with keto-friendly ranch dressing.

Nutrition Values (Per Serving)

- Calories: 125
- Fat: 7g
- Carbohydrates: 15g
- Protein: 2g

Cheesy Broccoli

(Prep time: 15 minutes\ Cook time: 8 minutes\ 2 servings)

Ingredients

- 1 small head of broccoli
- 1 Tbsp olive oil
- Juice from 1 lemon
- ¼ cup finely shredded parmesan cheese
- Pinch of salt, pepper

Directions

1. Rinse the broccoli. Pat dry. Dice into bite-size florets.
2. Place florets in Ziploc baggie.
3. Combine oil and lemon juice. Drizzle over florets.
4. Season with salt, pepper. Sprinkle cheese over florets.
5. Pre-heat fryer to 325°F. Lightly spray cook basket with non-stick Keto cooking spray.
6. Place florets in the fryer. Cook 8 minutes; shake at halfway point. (Want them slightly crunchy. Test after 5 minutes then every minute for desired crunch).
7. Transfer to platter. Seve with Keto-friendly dip.

Nutrition Values (Per Serving)

- Calories: 114
- Fat: 6g
- Carbohydrates: 10g
- Protein: 7g

Portobello Pizza

(Prep time: 10 minutes\ Cook time: 10 minutes\ 2 servings)

Ingredients

- 4 large portabella mushroom caps
- 3 Tbsp tomato sauce
- 3 Tbsp finely shredded mozzarella cheese
- Mini pepperoni slices

Directions

1. Remove stems, scoop out inside of mushrooms. Wipe them with a damp cloth. (Never wash mushrooms as it changes cooking consistency.)
2. Spray a light layer of oil over inside of mushroom.
3. Cover bottom of fryer with parchment paper. Spray light coating of oil on parchment.
4. Pre-heat fryer to 325°F. Lightly spray cook basket with non-stick Keto cooking spray.
5. Place in the fryer. Cook 5 minutes.
6. Spread a layer of tomato sauce on inside of mushroom. Top with pepperoni then cheese or cheese then pepperoni. Cook 5 minutes.
7. Transfer to platter. Garnish with fresh red pepper flakes.

Nutrition Values (Per Serving)

- Calories: 225
- Fat: 12g
- Carbohydrates: 16g
- Protein: 10g

Cheddar Bacon Croquettes

(Prep time: 10 minutes\ Cook time: 8 minutes\ 2 servings)

Ingredients

- 16 cubes sharp cheddar cheese
- 6 slices thin slice bacon
- 4 Tbsp flavorless oil
- 1 cup almond meal
- ½ tsp garlic powder
- ½ tsp onion powder
- ½ oregano
- Dash of salt, pepper
- 2 eggs
- 1 cup almond flour
- Garnish: fresh parsley

Directions

1. In a bowl, combine meal, garlic powder, onion powder, oregano, salt, pepper. Mix well.
2. Cut bacon slices in half. Wrap one half around the cheese from one side to the other, then alternate and wrap other half around cube; completely covering cube.
3. Pour the flour in a bowl. Beat the eggs in a separate bowl.
4. Dip wrapped cheese in flour, then egg, then seasoned meal, shake off excess. Place on a tray. Set tray in freezer 5 minutes to settle coating.
5. Pre-heat fryer to 390°F. Lightly spray cook basket with non-stick Keto cooking spray.
6. Place cubes in the fryer. Spray a light coating of oil on them. Cook 8 minutes.
7. Serve on a platter. Garnish with fresh parsley, side with Keto-friendly marinara sauce.

Nutrition Values (Per Serving)

- Calories: 333
- Fat: 26g
- Carbohydrates: 16g
- Protein: 5g

Crispy Shirataki Noodles

(Prep time: 5 minutes\ Cook time: 3 minutes\ 2 servings)

Ingredients

- 2 cups boiling water
- 1 Tbsp of Italian seasoning
- 1 Tbsp olive oil
- 2 cups Shirataki noodles
- Garnish: diced green onion, parmesan cheese

Directions

1. Pour boiling water over noodles. Allow to set 5 minutes.
2. Drain the water. Pat dry the noodles. Transfer to a bowl.
3. Spray a light coating of oil on the noodles. Season the noodles with italian seasoning, tossing to coat evenly.
4. Pre-heat fryer to 390°F. Lightly spray cook basket with non-stick Keto cooking spray.
5. Transfer noodles to the fryer. Cook 3 minutes, until crispy.
6. Serve in a bowl. Garnish with diced green onion, parmesan cheese.

Nutrition Values (Per Serving)

- Calories: 296
- Fat: 21g
- Carbohydrates: 16g
- Protein: 10g

Spinach Chips

(Prep time: 10 minutes\ Cook time: 2 minutes\ 2 servings)

Ingredients

- 1 bag baby spinach
- 2 Tbsp sesame oil
- Seasoning of choice; malt vinegar powder/salt, italian seasoning, cajun seasoning

Directions

1. Wash the spinach and dry thoroughly.
2. Lightly spray the spinach leaves with oil. Season with your choice of seasoning.
3. Pre-heat fryer to 375°F. Lightly spray cook basket with non-stick Keto cooking spray.
4. Place spinach chips in the fryer. Cook 2 minutes; shake, cook 1 more minute until crispy.
5. Transfer to platter. Allow to cool before eating.

Nutrition Values (Per Serving)

- Calories: 209
- Fat: 19g
- Carbohydrates: 3g
- Protein: 8g

Siracha Shrimp

(Prep time: 20 minutes\ Cook time: 6 minutes\ 2 servings)

Ingredients

- 20 shrimp, shelled, deveined
- 1 Tbsp siracha sauce
- 4 Tbsp corn starch
- 2 egg whites
- 3 Tbsp Panko bread crumbs
- 2 Tbsp flavorless oil

Directions

1. Rinse the shrimp. Pat dry. Place the shrimp in a bowl. Add the siracha sauce. Stir to coat evenly. Allow to marinate as you prepare other ingredients.
2. Three bowls: corn starch in one, egg whites in one, bread crumbs in one.
3. Dip shrimp in corn starch, then egg whites, then panko bread crumbs.
4. Line bottom of fryer with parchment paper.
5. Spray light coating of oil on parchment paper. Pre-heat fryer to 375°F.
6. Place shrimp in the fryer. Cook 3 minutes.
7. Turn the shrimp, spray with more oil. Cook 3 more minutes, until cooked thoroughly.
8. Serve on a platter. Side with cocktail sauce.

Nutrition Values (Per Serving)

- Calories: 270
- Fat: 9g
- Carbohydrates: 11g
- Protein: 9g

Daikon Fries

(Prep time: 10 minutes\ Cook time: 10 minutes\ 2 servings)

Ingredients

- 1 pound daikon
- 1 Tbsp olive oil
- 2 Tbsp almond meal
- ½ tsp of sage
- ½ tsp dried oregano
- Pinch of salt, pepper

Directions

1. Scrub but don't peel the daikon. Pat dry. Cut off most of end; leave small part to grab.
2. Coat daikon with light layer of oil.
3. Season almond meal with sage, dried oregano, salt, pepper. Use a wooden spoon to mesh it together. Dip daikon in seasoned meal.
4. Pre-heat fryer to 390°F. Lightly spray cook basket with non-stick Keto cooking spray.
5. Place daikon in the fryer. Cook 6 minutes.
6. Flip the daikon. Cook 4 more minutes.
7. Transfer to a platter. Serve with a Keto-friendly dipping sauce.

Nutrition Values (Per Serving)

- Calories: 43
- Fat: 2g
- Carbohydrates: 4g
- Protein: 2g

Egg Clouds

(Prep time: 8 minutes\ Cook time: 4 minutes\ 2 servings)

Ingredients

- 2 eggs

Directions

1. Separate the eggs; egg whites and egg yolks.
2. Whisk the egg whites until a strong peek forms.
3. Pre-heat fryer to 300°F. Lightly spray cook basket with non-stick Keto cooking spray.
4. Using a large spoon, gently dollop egg white in the fryer. (May have to cook in batches.)
5. Cook 2 minutes.
6. Whisk the yellow as the white cooks.
7. Open the fryer. Spoon egg yellow in middle of cooked egg white. Cook 2 minutes.
8. Transfer to a plate. Serve with brown toast.

Nutrition Values (Per Serving)

- Calories: 80
- Fat: 6g
- Carbohydrates: 0.3g
- Protein: 5.6g

Egg Soufflé

(Prep time: 8 minutes\ Cook time: 8 minutes\ 2 servings)

Ingredients

- 2 eggs
- 1 Tbsp heavy cream,
- 1 Tbsp dried parsley
- ¼ tsp ground chili powder
- ¼ tsp salt

Directions

1. In a bowl, combine the eggs, cream, parsley, chili powder, salt. Whisk briskly.
2. Pour mixture evenly between ramekins.
3. Pre-heat fryer to 300°F.
4. Place dishes in the fryer. Cook 8 minutes.
5. Remove from fryer. Allow to cool slightly.

Nutrition Values (Per Serving)

- Calories: 116
- Fat: 10g
- Carbohydrates: 0.9g
- Protein: 5.9g

Spam Fries

(Prep time: 8 minutes\ Cook time: 10 minutes\ 2 servings)

Ingredients

- 1 can of Spam
- 1 tsp olive oil

Directions

1. Slice the spam into french fry size.
2. Spread a light coating of oil over the fries.
3. Pre-heat fryer to 350°F. Lightly spray cook basket with non-stick Keto cooking spray.
4. Place them in the fryer. Cook 10 minutes; until golden brown.
5. Transfer to a platter. Serve with a Keto-friendly dipping sauce.

Nutrition Values (Per Serving)

- Calories: 116
- Fat: 10g
- Carbohydrates: 0.9g
- Protein: 5.9g

Buffalo Wings

(Prep time: 10 minutes\ Cook time: 16 minutes\ 2 servings)

Ingredients

- 12 chicken wings
- 3 Tbsp melted butter
- ¼ cup favorite hot sauce
- Pinch of salt

Directions

1. Rinse the wings. Pat them dry.
2. In a bowl, combine the melted butter, hot sauce, salt.
3. Add the wings to the bowl. Stir until evenly coated. Refrigerate 2 hours.
4. Line bottom of fryer with parchment paper. Spray parchment paper with oil.
5. Pre-heat fryer to 400°F. Spray wings with a light coating of oil as well.
6. Place them in the fryer. Cook 8 minutes. Flip the wings. Spray other side with light coating of oil. Cook 8 more minutes.
7. Transfer to a platter.

Nutrition Values (Per Serving)

- Calories: 468
- Fat: 32g
- Carbohydrates: 2g
- Protein: 42g

Stuffed Mushrooms

(Prep time: 5 minutes\ Cook time: 8 minutes\ 2 servings)

Ingredients

- 14 button mushrooms
- 1 Tbsp olive oil
- ¼ cup cream cheese
- 1 tsp chili powder
- 1 tsp cumin seeds
- Pinch of salt, pepper
- 1 Tbsp minced garlic
- ¼ cup parmesan cheese
- Garnish: Fresh parsley

Directions

1. Wipe the mushrooms using a damp cloth. Remove stems.
2. Dice the stems.
3. In a bowl, combine diced stems, cream cheese, chili powder, cumin seeds, minced garlic, salt, pepper. Stir well.
4. In a separate bowl, drizzle oil over the mushroom caps.
5. Pre-heat fryer to 350°F. Lightly spray cook basket with non-stick Keto cooking spray.
6. Place mushroom caps in the fryer. Cook 5 minutes.
7. Using 2 spoons, place a dollop of the cream cheese mixture in the mushroom caps. Top with a pinch of parmesan cheese.
8. Cook 3 minutes, until golden brown on top.
9. Transfer to a platter. Garnish with fresh parsley.

Nutrition Values (Per Serving)

- Calories: 143
- Fat: 9g
- Carbohydrates: 10g
- Protein: 6g

Keto-Friendly Bacon

(Prep time: 8 minutes\ Cook time: 10 minutes\ 2 servings)

Ingredients

- 10 slices of bacon
- ½ tsp dried oregano
- ½ tsp ground thyme
- Pinch of salt, pepper

Directions

1. In a bowl, combine the oregano, thyme, salt, pepper.
2. Season the bacon with the spice mixture.
3. Let the bacon rest 3 minutes.
4. Pre-heat fryer to 350°F. Lightly spray cook basket with non-stick Keto cooking spray.
5. Place the bacon in the fryer. Cook 5 minutes. Flip over. Cook 5 more minutes.
6. Transfer bacon to serving platter.

Nutrition Values (Per Serving)

- Calories: 323
- Fat: 23g
- Carbohydrates: 1.5g
- Protein: 28g

Cheese bites

(Prep time: 15 minutes\ Cook time: 6 minutes\ 2 servings)

Ingredients

- 4 cheese sticks; your choice, mozzarella, cheddar
- 2 Tbsp almond flour
- 1 egg white
- 2 Tbsp panko bread crumbs
- ¼ tsp oregano
- Pinch of salt, pepper
- Garnish: fresh parsley, marinara sauce

Directions

1. Dice the cheese sticks into bite-size pieces; 3 pieces per stick.
2. In a bowl, combine the bread crumbs, oregano, salt, pepper.
3. In a separate bowl, whisk the egg white slightly.
4. In another bowl, pour the flour.
5. Start with dipping the cheese in flour, then egg white, then bread crumb; can repeat for a crunchier coating. Place on a tray. Set tray in the freezer for 10 minutes.
6. Cover bottom of fryer with parchment paper. Spray parchment paper with oil.
7. Pre-heat fryer to 325°F.
8. Spray coated cheese with light layer of oil. Place in the fryer. Cook 3 minutes.
9. Flip cheese bites at halfway point. Spray light layer of oil on other side. Cook 3 minutes; until golden brown.
10. Transfer to platter. Garnish with parsley. Serve with marinara sauce.

Nutrition Values (Per Serving)

- Calories: 127
- Fat: 7g
- Carbohydrates: 16g
- Protein: 7g

Chicken Livers

(Prep time: 10 minutes\ Cook time: 10 minutes\ 2 servings)

Ingredients

- ½ pound chicken livers
- 2 Tbsp almond meal
- 4 Tbsp of butter
- ½ tsp dried cilantro
- ½ tsp onion powder
- Pinch of salt, pepper
- Garnish: diced green onion

Directions

1. Dice the chicken livers into small pieces. Pat them dry.
2. Melt the butter.
3. In a bowl, combine almond meal, cilantro, onion powder, salt, pepper. Mix.
4. Dip chicken livers in butter. Dip in the seasoning. Place on a tray. Freeze for 5 minutes.
5. Pre-heat fryer to 350°F. Lightly spray cook basket with non-stick Keto cooking spray.
6. Place in the fryer. Cook 10 minutes; shake at halfway point.
7. Transfer to platter. Garnish with diced green onion. Serve with a Keto-friendly sauce.

Nutrition Values (Per Serving)

- Calories: 173
- Fat: 10g
- Carbohydrates: 2.2g
- Protein: 9g

Fried Eggs

(Prep time: 10 minutes\ Cook time: 5 minutes\ 2 servings)

Ingredients

- 4 eggs
- 1 Tbsp butter
- Pinch of salt, pepper

Directions

1. Pre-heat fryer to 325°F. Add butter to the fryer.
2. Crack an egg in fryer. Season with salt and pepper.
3. Cook 5 minutes.
4. Transfer to a plate.

Nutrition Values (Per Serving)

- Calories: 164
- Fat: 8g
- Carbohydrates: 21g
- Protein: 3g

Grilled Cheese

(Prep time: 5 minutes\ Cook time: 10 minutes\ 1 serving)

Ingredients

- 2 slices Keto-friendly bread; almond flour bread
- 2 slices cheese of your choice
- 2 tsp butter

Directions

1. Pre-heat air fryer to 350°F.
2. Butter each slice of bread. Place slice of cheese between bread slices.
3. Place in the fryer. Cook 10 minutes; flip at halfway point.
4. Transfer to a plate.

Nutrition Values (Per Serving)

- Calories: 143
- Fat: 9g
- Carbohydrates: 10g
- Protein: 6g

Chicken Strips

(Prep time: 10 minutes\ Cook time: 12 minutes\ 2 servings)

Ingredients

- 2 boneless, skinless chicken breasts
- 1 Tbsp butter
- 2 Tbsp almond flour
- 2 egg whites
- 2 Tbsp panko bread crumbs
- 1 tsp paprika
- Pinch of salt, pepper
- Garnish: diced green onions

Directions

1. Rinse the chicken. Pat dry. Slice chicken into strips.
2. Pour the flour in a bowl. In a separate bowl, whisk the egg whites slightly.
3. Pour the bread crumbs in a bowl. Add the paprika, salt, pepper. Stir.
4. Dip chicken strips in the flour, then egg whites, then bread crumbs; repeat for a crunchier coating. Place on a tray. Set the tray in freezer for 5 minutes.
5. Cover bottom of fryer with parchment paper. Lightly spray parchment with oil.
6. Pre-heat fryer to 350°F.
7. Spray a light coating on the chicken strips. Place in the fryer. Cook 6 minutes. Flip over. Spray another light coating on other side. Cook another 6 minutes; until golden brown.
8. Transfer to serving platter. Garnish with diced green onion. Serve with Keto-friendly ranch dressing.

Nutrition Values (Per Serving)

- Calories: 40
- Fat: 3.9g
- Carbohydrates: 0.5g
- Protein: 1.2g

Brisket Bites

(Prep time: 15 minutes\ Cook time: 10 minutes\ 2 servings)

Ingredients

- ½ pound cooked pork brisket
- 6 thin slices of bacon
- 1 Tbsp apple cider vinegar
- 1 tsp turmeric
- Pinch of salt, pepper
- Toothpicks
- Garnish: fresh parsley

Directions

1. Dice the brisket into bite-size pieces.
2. In a bowl, combine the apple cider vinegar, turmeric, pepper, salt. Mix well.
3. Add the pork bites to the apple cider mix. Marinate 10 minutes.
4. Wrap the bites in sliced bacon. Secure with toothpicks.
5. Pre-heat fryer to 350°F. Lightly spray cook basket with non-stick Keto cooking spray.
6. Place in the fryer. Cook 5 minutes. Flip over. Cook 5 more minutes.
7. Transfer to plater. Garnish with parsley.

Nutrition Values (Per Serving)

- Calories: 239
- Fat: 13g
- Carbohydrates: 3g
- Protein: 26g

Zucchini Fries

(Prep time: 15 minutes\ Cook time: 10 minutes\ 2 servings)

Ingredients

- 2 large zucchini
- 2 Tbsp flour
- 2 egg whites
- ½ cup almond meal
- 2 Tbsp finely shred parmesan cheese
- ¼ tsp garlic powder
- Pinch of salt, pepper

Directions

1. Peel the zucchini. Slice in french fry size.
2. In a bowl, combine the almond meal, parmesan cheese, garlic powder, salt, pepper.
3. In a separate bowl, pour in the flour.
4. In another bowl, whisk the egg whites softly.
5. Dip the zucchini in flour, then egg whites, then the almond meal. Place on a tray. Set the tray in the freezer for 5 minutes.
6. Cover bottom of fryer with parchment paper. Lightly spray parchment with oil.
7. Pre-heat fryer to 350°F. Lightly spray cook basket with non-stick Keto cooking spray.
8. Place zucchini fries in the fryer. Cook 5 minutes.
9. Flip over. Spray with oil. Cook 5 more minutes.
10. Transfer to platter. Garnish with diced green onions. Serve with Keto-friendly ranch dressing.

Nutrition Values (Per Serving)

- Calories: 204
- Fat: 8g
- Carbohydrates: 14g
- Protein: 12g

Fried Okra

(Prep time: 8 minutes\ Cook time: 4 minutes\ 2 servings)

Ingredients

- 6 okra
- 1 Tbsp sesame oil
- ½ tsp of salt, pepper
- ¼ tsp garlic powder
- 1 whole egg
- Garnish: sesame seeds

Directions

1. Wash the okra. Dice in circles. Place the sliced okra in a large Ziploc bag.
2. In a bowl, whisk the egg. Dip the okra in the egg.
3. In a separate bowl, combine the garlic powder, salt, pepper. Season the okra. Place okra on a tray. Place tray in freezer 5 minutes.
4. Pre-heat fryer to 350°F. Lightly spray cook basket with non-stick Keto cooking spray.
5. Place okra in the fryer. Cook 4 minutes; shake at halfway point.
6. Transfer to platter. Garnish with sesame seeds.

Nutrition Values (Per Serving)

- Calories: 81
- Fat: 5g
- Carbohydrates: 7g
- Protein: 3g

Bacon Wrapped Jalapenos

(Prep time: 15 minutes\ Cook time: 10 minutes\ 2 servings)

Ingredients

- 6 slices thin slice bacon
- 6 jalapeno peppers
- 1 tsp olive oil

Directions

1. Wipe the jalapenos with a damp cloth.
2. You have the option here. Core the jalapenos, remove the seeds, or leave the seeds in. Either way, snip off each end.
3. Wrap a slice of bacon around the pepper. Lightly spray bacon wrapped pepper with oil.
4. Pre-heat fryer to 350°F. Lightly spray cook basket with non-stick Keto cooking spray.
5. Place peppers in the fryer. Cook 5 minutes. Flip over. Cook for 5 more minutes.
6. Transfer to platter. Serve with Keto-friendly dipping sauce.

Nutrition Values (Per Serving)

- Calories: 198
- Fat: 15g
- Carbohydrates: 2g
- Protein: 12g

Onion And Sage Stuffed Balls

(Prep time: 10 minutes\ Cook time: 15 minutes\ 2 servings)

Ingredients

- ¼ cup meat sauce
- ½ small onion
- ½ tsp fresh sage
- ½ tsp garlic puree
- 2 Tbsp flavorless oil
- 3 Tbsp almond meal
- Pinch of salt, pepper

Directions

1. In a bowl, combine the ingredients. Stir until combined.
2. Using a small spoon, measure out an amount to create bite-size balls.
3. Lightly spray the balls with oil. Dip in the almond meal. Place on a tray. Set tray in freezer for 5 minutes.
4. Pre-heat fryer to 350°F. Lightly spray cook basket with non-stick Keto cooking spray.
5. Place balls in the fryer. Cook 10 minutes; flip at halfway point.
6. Transfer to platter. Side with a Keto-friendly marinara.

Nutrition Values (Per Serving)

- Calories: 257
- Fat: 20g
- Carbohydrates: 11g
- Protein: 9g

Warm Broccoli Salad

(Prep time: 10 minutes\ Cook time: 5 minutes\ 2 servings)

Ingredients

- 1 large head of broccoli
- 1 Tbsp sesame oil
- 4 slices of bacon, cooked, crumbled
- 1 Tbsp chives
- 1 Tbsp apple cider vinegar
- 1 tsp flax seed

Directions

1. Dice the broccoli into bite-size florets.
2. Sprinkle the florets with a light coating of oil.
3. Pre-heat fryer to 350°F. Lightly spray cook basket with non-stick Keto cooking spray.
4. Place in the fryer. Cook 6 minutes.
5. As they cook, in a large bowl, combine the crumbled bacon, chives, flax seed. Set aside.
6. Once broccoli is cooked, transfer to the bowl with other ingredients.
7. Drizzle apple cider vinegar over ingredients. Stir well.

Nutrition Values (Per Serving)

- Calories: 217
- Fat: 15g
- Carbohydrates: 6g
- Protein: 13g

Egg Tarts

(Prep time: 10 minutes\ Cook time: 10 minutes\ 2 servings)

Ingredients

- 2 egg whites
- Handful baby spinach leaves
- 1 small tomato, diced
- 2 Tbsp finely shredded parmesan cheese, or any other choice
- 1 tsp butter
- Pinch of salt, pepper

Directions

1. Dice the tomato. In a bowl, whisk the egg whites. Add the tomato, spinach, cheese, salt, pepper to the bowl. Stir together.
2. Lightly grease 2 ramekin dishes. Divide the mixture between the two dishes.
3. Pre-heat fryer to 350°F. Place ramekins in the fryer. Cook 10 minutes.
4. Serve with cooked vegetables.

Nutrition Values (Per Serving)

- Calories: 204
- Fat: 16g
- Carbohydrates: 12g
- Protein: 5g

Parmesan Sticks

(Prep time: 10 minutes\ Cook time: 8 minutes\ 2 servings)

Ingredients

- 10 strips parmesan cheese
- 1 egg
- ½ cup heavy cream
- 4 Tbsp almond flour
- ¼ tsp pepper

Directions

1. Cut the parmesan cheese into french fry size.
2. In a bowl, whisk the egg. Add heavy cream, pepper, almond flour. Stir well.
3. Dip the cheese into batter. Place on a tray. Set tray in freezer 30 minutes.
4. Pre-heat fryer to 350°F. Lightly spray cook basket with non-stick Keto cooking spray.
5. Place cheese sticks in the fryer. Cook 8 minutes.
6. Transfer to serving plate. Serve with a Keto-friendly dipping sauce.

Nutrition Values (Per Serving)

- Calories: 398
- Fat: 30g
- Carbohydrates: 6g
- Protein: 28g

Chapter 8: Desserts

Apricot And Blackberry Crumble

(Prep time: 10 minutes\ Cook time: 20 minutes\ 2 servings)

Ingredients

- 2 apricots, peeled, diced
- ½ cup fresh blackberries
- 2 Tbsp lemon juice
- ½ cup almond flour
- 1 tsp ground cinnamon
- 1 Tbsp brown sugar
- Pinch of salt
- 5 Tbsp cold butter, diced
- Keto-friendly whip cream or heavy cream

Directions

1. In a large bowl, combine diced apricots and blackberries. Drizzle lemon juice over fruits.
2. In another bowl, add the almond flour, ground cinnamon, brown sugar, salt. Stir.
3. Add the butter. Using 2 knives or pastry cutter, combine to a crumble consistency.
4. Grease individual baking dishes, spoon in fruit mixture. Top with crumble.
5. Pre-heat fryer to 350°F.
6. Transfer dishes to the fryer. Cook 20 minutes.
7. Remove from the fryer. Allow to cool slightly. Top with Keto-friendly cream.

Nutrition Values (Per Serving)

- Calories: 382
- Fat: 30g
- Carbohydrates: 18g
- Protein: 5g

Fried Pineapple

(Prep time: 10 minutes\ Cook time: 8 minutes\ 2 servings)

Ingredients

- 2 Tbsp shredded coconut
- 2 Tbsp agave nectar
- 1 Tbsp lime juice
- 1 small pineapple

Directions

1. Remove the skin and crown. Core the pineapple.
2. Slice in circles. In a bowl, combine agave nectar and lime juice. Stir well.
3. Cover bottom of fryer with parchment paper. Lightly spray parchment with oil.
4. Pre-heat fryer to 350°F.
5. Place pineapple in the fryer. Sprinkle coconut on one side of pineapple. Cook 4 minutes. Flip over. Add more coconut. Cook 4 minutes, until golden brown.
6. Transfer to platter. Allow to cool before eating.

Nutrition Values (Per Serving)

- Calories: 300
- Fat: 22g
- Carbohydrates: 14g
- Protein: 12g

Toasted Marshmallows

(Prep time: 5 minutes\ Cook time: 4 minutes\ 2 servings)

Ingredients

- 1 tsp butter
- 6 large marshmallows
- Keto-friendly peanut butter

Directions

1. Lightly grease a pyrex dish with butter. Place the large marshmallows in the dish so they are touching.
2. Pre-heat fryer to 350°F. Cook 4 minutes.
3. Drizzle peanut butter over toasted marshmallows.

Nutrition Values (Per Serving)

- Calories: 204
- Fat: 16g
- Carbohydrates: 12g
- Protein: 5g

Banana Fritters

(Prep time: 10 minutes\ Cook time: 8 minutes\ 2 servings)

Ingredients

- ¼ cup almond flour
- 2 large bananas
- 1 tsp salt
- 1 tsp sesame oil
- Pinch of ground cinnamon
- 1 Tbsp water

Directions

1. Peel the banana. Dice into bite-size pieces.
2. In a bowl, combine the flour, salt, sesame oil. Add 1 tablespoon of water. Stir until combined in a smooth batter. (If too dry, add a bit more water until smooth but not too thick batter.)
3. Dip banana in batter. Set on a tray. Place tray in freezer for 10 minutes.
4. Cover bottom of fryer with parchment paper. Spray parchment with oil.
5. Pre-heat fryer to 350°F.
6. Place bananas in fryer. Spray bananas with a light coating of oil. Cook 4 minutes, flip over, spray oil on other side. Cook 4 more minutes; until golden brown.
7. Transfer to a platter. Dust with powdered sugar.

Nutrition Values (Per Serving)

- Calories: 242
- Fat: 9g
- Carbohydrates: 18g
- Protein: 5g

Vanilla Custard

(Prep time: 10 minutes\ Cook time: 20 minutes\ 2 servings)

Ingredients

- 5 eggs
- ½ cup cream cheese, room temperature
- ½ cup almond milk, room temperature
- 1 tsp vanilla extract
- 2 Tbsp Erythritol
- 1 tsp butter

Directions

1. In a bowl, beat the eggs with a mixer. Add the cream cheese, water, vanilla extract, Erythritol. Beat 2 minutes.
2. Lightly grease 2 ramekins with butter. Divide the batter between the ramekins.
3. Cover bottom of the fryer with parchment paper.
4. Pre-heat fryer to 350°F.
5. Place ramekins in the fryer. Cook 20 minutes.
6. Remove from the fryer. Allow to cool before eating. Serve with fresh berries.

Nutrition Values (Per Serving)

- Calories: 183
- Fat: 15g
- Carbohydrates: 15g
- Protein: 10g

Mini chocolate cake

(Prep time: 15 minutes\ Cook time: 5 minutes\ 2 servings)

Ingredients

- ¼ cup flour
- ¼ cup sugar
- 2 Tbsp cocoa powder
- ⅛ tsp baking soda
- ⅛ tsp salt
- 3 Tbsp milk
- 2 Tbsp flavorless oil
- 1 Tbsp water
- ¼ tsp vanilla extract

Directions

1. In a bowl, combine the flour, sugar, cocoa powder, baking soda, salt. Stir.
2. In a separate bowl, combine the milk, oil, water, vanilla. Stir.
3. Add the dry ingredients to the liquid. Stir until smooth.
4. Lightly grease 2 ramekins or small (heat resistant) mugs.
5. Divide batter evenly between dishes.
6. Cover bottom of fryer with parchment paper. Pre-heat fryer to 325°F.
7. Place ramekins in the fryer. Cook 5 minutes.
8. Remove from fryer. Allow to cool. Serve with fresh berries, whip cream.

Nutrition Values (Per Serving)

- Calories: 403
- Fat: 30g
- Carbohydrates: 6.9g
- Protein: 4g

Conclusion

I would like to thank you again for reading the book.
I hope this book has been helpful and you found the information useful.
Keep in mind that you are not only limited to the recipes provided in this book. Keep exploring until you unlock the true potential of your Air Fryer and Ketogenic regime. Stay safe and healthy.

Made in the USA
Columbia, SC
31 December 2018